The Sirtfood Diet

The Easy Beginners Guide for Fast Weight Loss and Burn Fat. Activate Your Metabolism Through the Super Power of Sirtfoods

CATHERINE MILLER

Copyright @ 2020 Catherine Miller - All rights reserved

This book is written with the sole purpose of providing relevant information on a specific topic for which every reasonable effort has been made to ensure that it is both accurate and reasonable. Nevertheless, by purchasing this book, you consent to the fact that the author, as well as the publisher, are in no way experts on the topics contained herein, regardless of any claims as such that may be made within. As such, any suggestions or recommendations that are made within are made so purely for entertainment value. It is recommended that you always consult a professional prior to undertaking any of the advice or techniques discussed within.

This is a legally binding declaration that is considered both valid and fair by both the Committee of Publishers Association and the American Bar Association and should be considered as legally binding within the United States.

The reproduction, transmission, and duplication of any of the content found herein, including any specific or extended information, will be done as an illegal act regardless of the end form the information ultimately takes. This includes copied versions of the work, both physical, digital, and audio, unless express consent of the Publisher is provided beforehand. Any additional rights reserved.

Furthermore, the information that can be found within the pages described forthwith shall be considered both accurate and truthful when it comes to the recounting of facts. As such, any use, correct or incorrect, of the provided information will render the Publisher free of responsibility as to the actions taken outside of their direct purview. Regardless, there are zero scenarios where the original author or the Publisher can be deemed liable in any fashion for any damages or hardships that may result from any of the information discussed herein.

Additionally, the information in the following pages is intended only for informational purposes and should thus be thought of as universal. As befitting its nature, it is presented without assurance regarding its prolonged validity or interim quality. Trademarks that are mentioned are done without written consent and can in no way be considered an endorsement from the trademark holder.

TABLE OF CONTENTS

Introduction 7
CHAPTER 1: HOW DOES THE SIRT DIET WORK 9
    Diet opinions Sirt 14
    Testimonials 14
CHAPTER 2 - THE TOP SIRT FOODS 17
    Buckwheat 19
    Capers 22
    Celery 26
    Chilli pepper – Bird's-eye chilli 29
    Curly kale 34
    Cocoa 39
    Coffee 43
    Extra virgin olive oil 45
    Lovage 49
    Matcha Green Tea 53
    Medjool dates 57
    Parsley 59
    Red chicory 62
    Red Onion 65
    Red wine 67
    Rocket Salad 70
    Soy 75
    Strawberries 77
    Turmeric 79
    Walnuts 81

CHAPTER 3 - THE GREEN JUICE 87
Options 89
CHAPTER 4 – DIET PLAN 91
The First Phase 91
The Second Phase 93
CHAPTER 5: THE FIRST PHASE: 7 POUNDS IN 7 DAYS 95
7-Day Meal Plan 95
Day 1 95
Recipe 1 - Prawns with buckwheat 96
Or Recipe 2- Turkey with cauliflower couscous 97
Day 2 99
Recipe 3 - Chicken with red onion and kale 100
Or Recipe 4 – Vegetable and buckwheat soup 102
Day 3 104
Recipe 5 - Pasta with smoked salmon with chilli and rocket 105
Or Recipe 6 – Buckwheat and tofu salad 106
Day 4 108
Recipe 7 - Chocolate Tartufini Sirt 109
Or Recipe 8 - Waldorf Salad 110
Day 5 112
Recipe 9 - Buckwheat pancakes with strawberries and chocolate 113
Or Recipe 10 - Pumpkin soup 115
Day 6 117
Recipe 11 - Chicken breast with walnut and parmesan pesto and red onion 118
Or Recipe 12 - Meat and chilli 119
Day 7 121
Recipe 13 - Pizza Sirt 121
Or Recipe 14 - Buckwheat pasta salad 124

CHAPTER 6: THE SECOND PHASE: MAINTENANCE 125

  RECIPES 125

    Recipe 15 - Buckwheat and broccoli with chickpeas 125

    Recipe 16 - Buckwheat meatballs. 126

    Recipe 17 - Cabbage and buckwheat fritters 128

    Recipe 18 - Buckwheat salad with artichokes 129

    Recipe 19 - Pasta with rocket salad and linseed 131

    Recipe 20 - Rocket and strawberry salad 132

    Recipe 21 – Sirt Meat & chilli 133

    Recipe 22 - Sirt Eggs 134

    Recipe 23 – Sirt Yogurt 135

    Recipe 24 – Sirt pita bread 136

    Recipe 25 – Sirt Omelette 137

    Recipe 26 – Red bean sauce with baked potato 138

    Recipe 27 – Tuna turkey 139

    Recipe 28 - Stew with sirtfood 141

    Recipe 29 – Curly kale with sweet potatoes 142

    Recipe 30 – Buckwheat pasta with zucchini and cherry tomatoes 143

    Recipe 31 – Chicken curry with potatoes and cabbage 144

    Recipe 32 – Cabbage and buckwheat soup 146

    Recipe 33 – Pasta with red chicory and walnuts 147

    Recipe 34 - Cabbage and red chicory flan 147

    Recipe 35 - Red chicory and kale salad 149

    Recipe 36 - Salmon and rocket fusilli 150

    Recipe 37 - Cabbage soup and chickpeas with turmeric 151

    Recipe 38 - Strawberries in salad 152

    Recipe 39 - Turmeric chicken 153

    Recipe 40 - Pork tenderloin with apricots 154

CHAPTER 7: QUESTIONS & ANSWERS 157
Conclusion 161
Conversions *162*
   Grams to Ounces *162*
   Celsius to Fahrenheit...*164*

Introduction

Thank you for buying this book, in which we will talk about a revolutionary method of nutrition that allows you to lose weight quickly and effectively. It is possible; thanks to the consumption of certain foods that have the power to accelerate metabolism.

Not surprisingly, more and more often, we hear about the Sirtfood diet, a diet based on foods rich in sirtuins, proteins with enzymatic action that can activate the metabolism and help lose weight.

The success of this diet is due to the speed with which it would be able to lose weight: 7 pounds in 7 days! An exceptional result when you think of the weight loss as due to the consumption of specific foods that have the power to activate and accelerate the metabolism and, therefore, burn excess fat, stressing the drop in body weight.

After reading this book, nothing will be hidden from you any more about these foods because you will acquire a thorough knowledge that will allow you to use them whenever you want.

Members are required to follow a fourteen-day plan, which includes a reduction in calorie consumption and the consumption of "Sirtfood green juices."

In the first part of this diet, you will be accompanied by hand. In fact, in this book, I have included a 7-day diet plan, complete with recipes. In the first phase, you can choose between two recipes proposed, according to your taste.

At the end of the first week, you should already lose 7 pounds; also thanks to the loss of excess liquids.

In this book, you will find many new recipes prepared with foods rich in sirtuin. You can focus on a more balanced and sirtfood-rich diet. It will allow you to achieve the extraordinary goal of a healthier and fitter body.

It only takes a little while to get started, and just seven days to evaluate your first progress. Don't wait any longer; take charge of your life and make it great!

Enjoy!

CHAPTER 1: HOW DOES THE SIRT DIET WORK

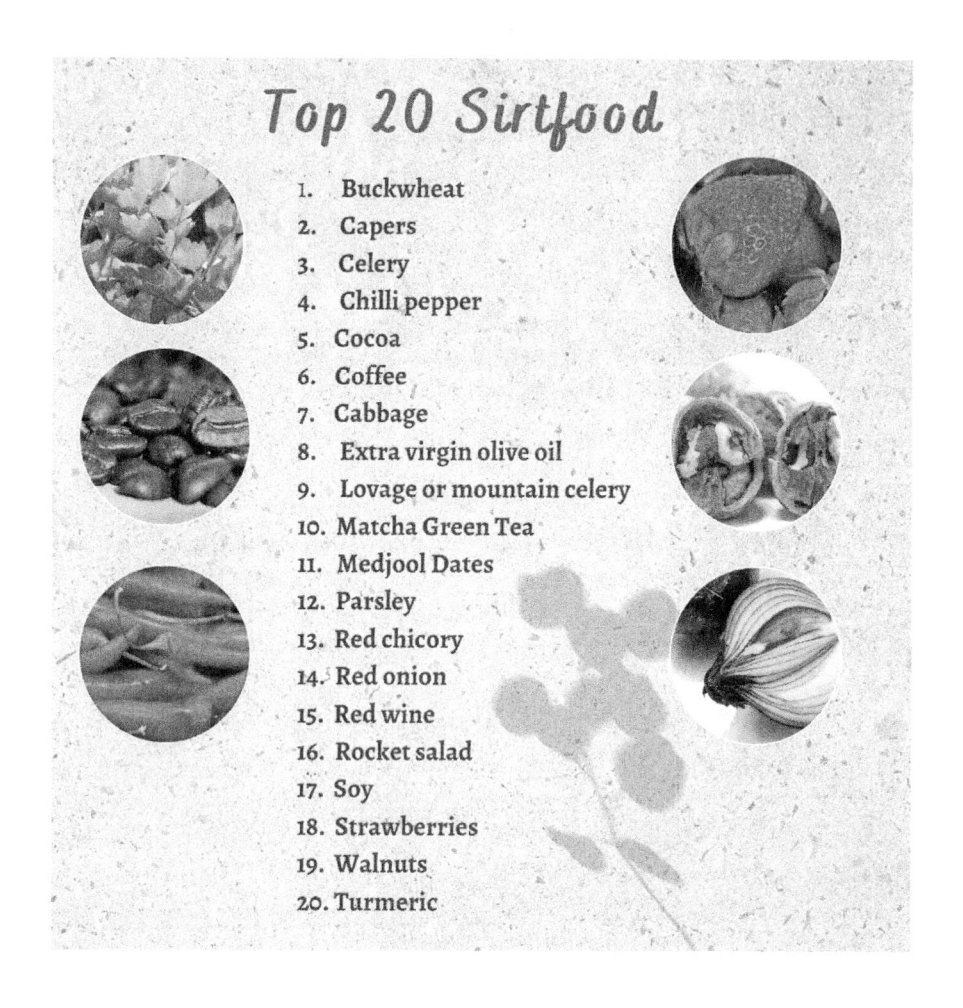

Top 20 Sirtfood

1. Buckwheat
2. Capers
3. Celery
4. Chilli pepper
5. Cocoa
6. Coffee
7. Cabbage
8. Extra virgin olive oil
9. Lovage or mountain celery
10. Matcha Green Tea
11. Medjool Dates
12. Parsley
13. Red chicory
14. Red onion
15. Red wine
16. Rocket salad
17. Soy
18. Strawberries
19. Walnuts
20. Turmeric

The Sirtfood diet presents an entirely new diet, based on a group of nutrients capable of activating a family of genes already existing in each of us: sirtuins.

Our cells build seven different sirtuins (SIRT1 - SIRT7) that perform a variety of functions. Some bind to proteins in the cytoplasm and mitochondria and are involved in regulating a wide range of processes, from metabolism to neurodegeneration, and others control the transcription of genes. The fact is that the effect of sirtuins is so profound that they are called "super metabolic regulators." Sirtuins affect our ability to burn fat, mood, and the mechanisms that regulate longevity.

It has long been known in the scientific world that these genes are activated by calorie restriction, fasting, and physical activity. The activation of sirtuins by certain foods produces the same beneficial effects as fasting without the disadvantages, while naturally activating the metabolism.

Developed by nutritionists Aidan Goggins and Glen Matten, the sirtfoods diet prefers 20 foods (sirtfoods) rich in particular proteins, sirtuins. They can stimulate the metabolism and activate the "lean gene," which is combined with meat and fish.They should be consumed every day while drastically reducing the number of carbohydrates and the number of total daily calories.

These include dark chocolate (at least 85% cocoa) due to the presence of epicatechin, but also red wine, which is the original sirtfood, and the one from which the research behind this diet started. Its resveratrol content, together with piceatannol, are the key activators of sirtuin. Other activating nutrients are caffeic acid and chlorogenic acid contained in coffee. Then we have strawberries, onion, soy, parsley, cabbage, extra virgin olive oil, Matcha green tea, buckwheat, turmeric, walnuts, rocket, blueberries, capers, red chicory, tofu, chilli, and dates. These foods should be combined according to specific predefined menus, to stimulate the metabolism and lose weight without interfering with muscle mass.

What does the diet involve?

The diet is carried out in two stages. Phase one of three days that limits calories to 1,000 each day, consisting of three green juices and a sirtfood approved dinner.

Phase two lasts four days and increases the daily allocation by 1,500 calories per day with two green juices and two dinners.

After these phases, there is a support plan that does not focus on calories, but rather on reasonable portions, even dinners and topping up nearly with fish food. The 14-day maintenance plan highlights three meals, one green juice, and a couple of sirtfood snacks. Similarly, members are invited to finish 30 minutes of activity five days a week per government proposal, but this is not the main focus of the agreement.

But what are these "miracle foods"? Below we list some of them, but in the next chapters, we will analyze them all

The most basic ten include:
- Red wine
- Cocoa
- Celery

- Chilli pepper, especially birth's eye chilli
- Cabbage, especially curly kale
- Coffee
- Extra virgin olive oil
- Matcha Green Tea
- Red onion
- Walnuts

Over the last few years, fasting diets have become very popular. Indeed, studies show that by fasting - i.e., with a moderate daily calorie restriction or by practicing a more radical but less frequent intermittent fasting, you can expect to lose about six kilos in six months and substantially reduce the risk of contacting certain diseases. When fasting, the reduction of energy reserves activates the so-called "lean gene," which causes several positive changes. The accumulation of fat is interrupted, and the body blocks normal growth processes and enters into "survival" mode. The fat is burned faster, and the genes that repair and rejuvenate the cells are activated. As a result, we lose weight and increase our resistance to disease. All this, however, comes at a price. Lower energy intake leads to hunger, irritability, fatigue, and loss of muscle mass. And the problem is precisely this with fasting diets: when they are followed correctly they work, but they make us feel so bad that we can't respect them. The question, then, is this: is it possible to achieve the same results without having to impose that drastic drop in calories and without, therefore, suffering the negative consequences? At this point, we just have to introduce you to the Sirt foods, a group of newly discovered foods. Sirt foods are particularly rich in exceptional nutrients, able to activate the same genes of thinness that are stimulated by fasting. These genes are sirtuins. They became famous, thanks to a significant study conducted in 2003, during which scientists analyzed a particular substance, resveratrol, present in the skin of black grapes, red wine, and yeast, which would produce the same effects as calorie restriction without the need to decrease energy intake. Later, researchers discovered that other substances present in red wine have a similar impact, which would explain the benefits of consuming this drink and why those who consume it gain less weight. This fact naturally stimulated the search for other foods containing a high concentration of these nutrients, capable of producing such a beneficial effect in the body, and little by little, studies discovered different ones. While some are almost unknown, such as lovage, a herb that is now very little used in cooking, the vast majority are well known and widely used foods, such as extra virgin olive oil, red onions, parsley, chilli pepper, kale, strawberries, capers, tofu, cocoa, green tea, and even coffee.

Diet opinions Sirt

The Sirt diet divides nutritionists into two factions: supporters and opponents.

Supporters consider the Sirt diet to be an excellent slimming diet, easy to follow, and that keeps the promised results.

Those against compare the Sirt diet to a lightning diet, as they believe that the sudden weight loss is only due to the drastic reduction in heat in the first three days.

From our point of view, we can say that the Sirt diet, given its ease of implementation, can be taken into consideration without too many doubts. The foods allowed are healthy and nutritious, and among the Sirt foods, some foods satisfy the palate (such as dark chocolate) that lightens the fatigue of a diet.

Testimonials

The singer Adele

The most famous one is undoubtedly the singer Adele, who lost 30 kg in 12 months. The secret? The Sirt Diet. It is revealed by the international media, like the Daily Mail and the New York Post.

When Grammy Award-winning singer Adele discovered her incredible 40kg weight loss earlier this year, those who were ready to invite 2020 with new health and wellness goals were eager to find out what her mystery was.

Top model Lorraine Pascale

A fierce supporter of the Sirt diet is a former supermodel, now writer and celebrity chef on Anglo-Saxon TV, Lorraine Pascale, who says: "We all know that eating can be expensive. The beauty of Sirt foods is that many of them are already on our table every day. They are accessible and can be easily introduced into our diet."

"I wanted the waistline to fit my wedding dress."

Jadis, a 32-year-old marketing manager, was unhappy with her waistline and wanted to look suitable for her upcoming wedding. "A lot of people in my family have diabetes, so I always knew how to watch my weight, but I couldn't throw down the extra pounds, which my wedding dress would have put even more emphasis on." Following the Sirt diet, Jadis lost 7 pounds in 7 days and gained muscle mass, although she hadn't been exercising at the time.

"I was a housewife with two kids and too much extra weight."

Kate didn't like the extra pounds built up during pregnancy. She couldn't lose weight. By the end of the "trial" week on the Sirt diet, Kate had lost ten pounds. Her body fat percentage had dropped from 25 to 22 percent, allowing her to fall into the "fit" category as she wished.

The busy, stressed-out entrepreneur

Devoted to working and beyond the threshold of obesity, James tried the Sirt diet because, having diabetes in his family, he was worried he might get sick too. After seven days of dieting, he had lost 7 pounds. Even though he was still obese, it was the necessary starting point to make more radical changes. He understood that gaining weight was not inevitable and that he could remedy it. Another piece of good news: his blood glucose levels, which had reached prediabetes levels, had fallen substantially.

David Haye, former heavyweight champion

"Sirt foods have been a revelation in my diet. Introducing them allowed me to achieve a previously unimaginable body composition and well-being, and to prepare my return to the ring after a severe shoulder injury. If anyone asks me my number one rule of fitness, my answer is to adopt the Sirt Diet.

CHAPTER 2 - THE TOP SIRT FOODS

Millions of people in the world follow a diet every year, but only less than 1% of them will manage to make their weight loss permanent.

As nutritional medicine experts, we have never been a fan of diets. That is until we discovered sirtfoods.

These foods are rich in particular nutrients that promote the production of sirtuin, a protein that can activate the so-called "lean gene" faster than our bodies would typically do.

Here is a list of 20 foods that can help to "wake up" and regulate our metabolism, thanks to this diet.

The TOP Sirtfoods

1. Buckwheat
2. Capers
3. Celery
4. Chilli pepper, especially the bird's-eye chilli
5. Cocoa
6. Coffee
7. Cabbage
8. Extra virgin olive oil
9. Lovage or mountain celery
10. Matcha Green Tea
11. Medjool Dates
12. Parsley
13. Red chicory
14. Red onion
15. Red wine
16. Rocket salad
17. Soy
18. Strawberries
19. Walnuts
20. Turmeric

Buckwheat

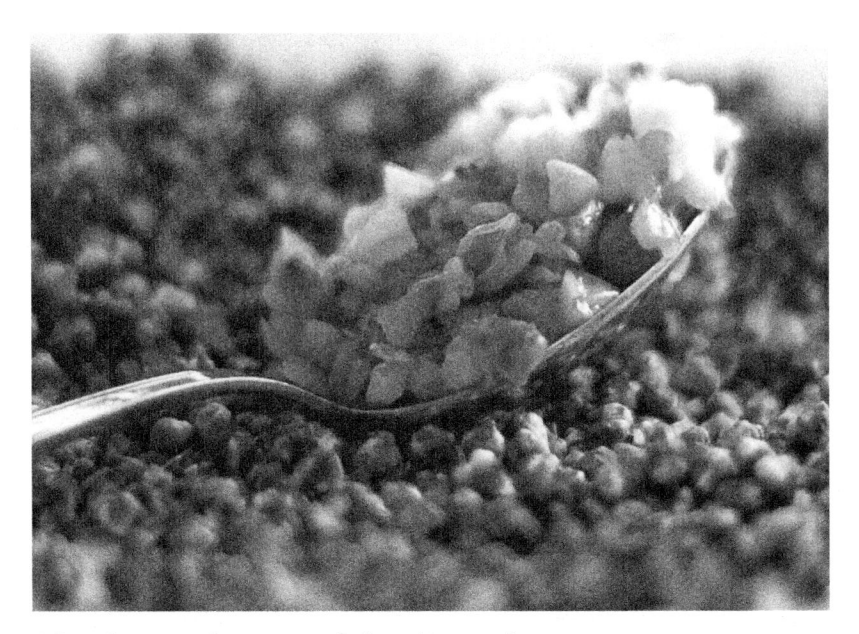

Nutrient activators of sirtuin: rutin.

Buckwheat is extremely popular in Japan, and tradition has it that when Buddhist monks traveled long distances in the mountains, all they took with them to produce food was a pot and a bag of buckwheat. This food was enough to feed them for weeks.

Buckwheat is a source of minerals such as iron, zinc, and selenium. Its seeds contain 18% protein, with a bio-absorbability value of over 90%. They contain essential amino acids, among which we find mainly lysine, threonine, and tryptophan. It is also a source of antioxidants, such as rutin and tannins. In particular, rutin is an activator of sirtuin; it tones the walls of capillary vessels to reduce the risk of bleeding. It is also considered beneficial for people suffering from hypertension or chronic venous insufficiency, as it helps to improve microcirculation. Its D-chiro-inositol content, linked to insulin production, makes it interesting for the treatment of diabetes.

Scientific research is investigating this aspect in its studies, which also concerns the use of buckwheat to lower cholesterol due to the presence of a protein able to bind firmly to it.

Buckwheat contains no gluten. This characteristic makes the consumption of both buckwheat beans and buckwheat flour suitable for people who have celiac disease and gluten intolerance.

In the natural diet, buckwheat is considered a cereal suitable for consumption, especially during the winter season, because of its remineralizing and fortifying properties, and because it can provide a lot of energy to our body. Its consumption is also recommended during breast-feeding and growth of children, as it favors the development and protection of the circulatory system in these delicate phases of life. The consumption of buckwheat can be useful for those suffering from high blood pressure or who need to keep cholesterol under control. Its use is not only recommended for those who have to avoid gluten for health reasons, but for all those who wish to bring more variety to their diet. It is recommended, especially in cases of tiredness and fatigue, to regain energy and to provide the body with the substances it needs to regenerate, such as amino acids and mineral salts.

Buckwheat is a food with no particular contraindications. The only aspect to keep in mind is any allergy or intolerance to this product. If you are likely to consume buckwheat during pregnancy, it is better to ask your doctor about it.

***

Capers

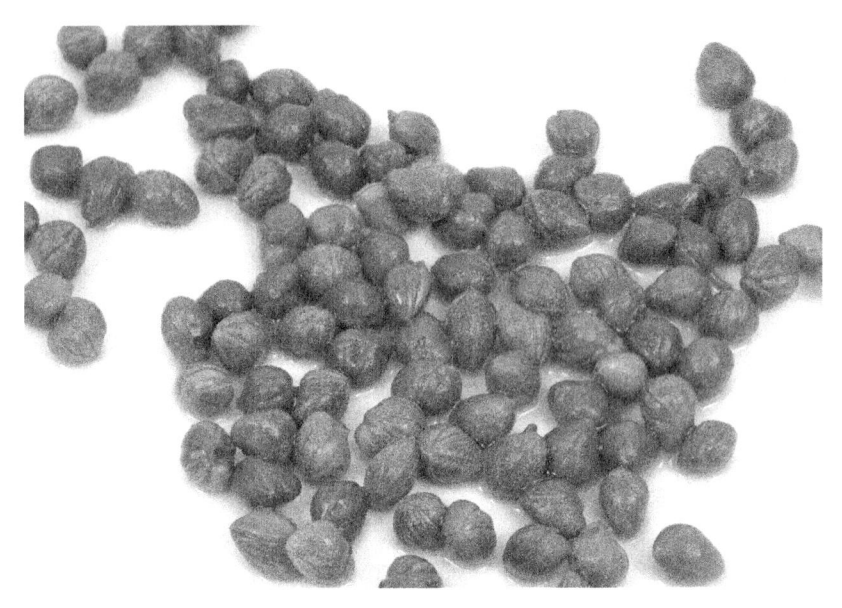

- Sirtuin activator nutrients: kaempferol and quercetin.

Capers are not fruits, but flower buds. The caper plant is widespread throughout the Mediterranean area and is rich in nutrients that promote the production of sirtuin.
All the benefits of capers:

1. Antitumoral and anti-inflammatories
Thanks to the large amount of quercetin, which we have seen to be a natural antioxidant. This food has an anti-inflammatory function, and quercetin itself is now being studied for its hypothetical anti-tumor properties.

These plant foods are also a good source of vitamin E that helps cells maintain their integrity. One study, carried out in 2014, established that capers contain powerful anti-tumor properties

2. Treatment of hemorrhoids
Roots of his plant produce an oily tincture. It is used for the treatment of hemorrhoids and inflammation of the mouth.

3. Immune System
Capers can strengthen the immune system. Studies show that caper extracts increase the activity of phagocytes. According to recent research in 2016, those who consume these plants certainly have a more efficient immune system.

4. Ultraviolet rays
According to a 2002 study, these plants contain compounds with properties that protect the skin from ultraviolet rays that can be dangerous to health, causing skin cancers such as melanoma. They also reduce redness and erythema caused by prolonged exposure to sunlight.

5. Moisturize the skin
Regular intake of capers benefits the skin. They moisturize the skin and provide relief in case of dryness.

6. Stimulants

Capers are recognized as stimulant properties that are especially beneficial to the appetite and digestive process.

7. Anti Allergic
A recent study has shown that this plant owns substances with properties able to combat certain types of skin allergy.

8. Lowers cholesterol
Rutin helps reduce blood cholesterol levels. It works mainly in obese people and inhibits the formation of dangerous plaques in the arteries. This has benefits for the cardiovascular system. The plant shoots also contain a substance that helps to reduce LDL cholesterol, niacin.

9. Diabetes
They are a useful food for people with diabetes. Research has shown that this plant contains substances that help reduce blood sugar levels. Their consumption also improves the functioning of the liver in people with diabetes without having side effects on the kidneys.

9. Weight Loss
Capers have good fiber content and low caloric intake. This combination is perfect for those who want to lose weight easily. To achieve this, however, it is necessary to introduce them naturally into your diet.

10. Allergies

It has been shown that the Extracts of *Capparis Spinosa* have anti-allergic properties. Capers contain substances with antihistamine effects, and others that control mast cells; compounds that lead to allergic reactions.

***

Celery

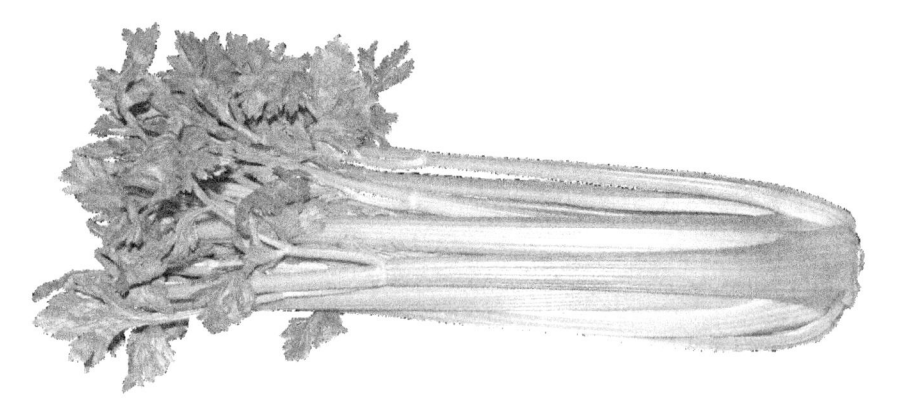

- Sirtuin activator nutrients: apigenin and luteolin.

There are two types of celery: white and green. Celery bleaching is a technique that was created to attenuate the particularly strong flavor of this vegetable, but it also compromises its ability to activate the production of sirtuin. The most nutritious parts of green celery are the heart and leaves.

Now let's see what all the benefits of this vegetable are.

1. <u>Celery, laxative properties</u>: it acts as a powerful laxative because it has large amounts of fiber, which works like a sponge that collects waste from the intestinal walls to make the stool flow much more quickly. Consuming it can eliminate this discomfort effortlessly and naturally.
2. <u>It promotes weight loss</u>: its composition is mostly water, almost 95%. Celery is one of the lightest vegetables that exist, especially for those who want to lose extra pounds. For every 100 grams, celery has only 16 calories, so we

can confirm that it is one of the vegetable foods with the lowest calorie content and is indicated for people suffering from obesity problems.

3. <u>Celery, diuretic properties</u>: this product has been found to contain selenium, limonene, and asparagine, i.e., oils that work as stimulants for optimal kidney activity; as well as potassium and sodium. It contributes to the process of removing excess fluid in the body.

4. <u>Inflammatory processes</u>: it is highly recommended in diseases such as asthma, arthritis, bronchitis, and even gout. You can take celery as an infusion (celery juice is delicious) or simply incorporate it into your daily diet.

5. <u>It prevents stomach and colon cancer</u>: Celery contains a group of components that have an anticarcinogenic effect, and a diet that includes a significant amount of celery can help as protection against stomach cancer and cancer of the digestive system.

6. <u>It improves kidney function</u>: not only is it useful to prevent the formation of kidney stones, but it also naturally stimulates the adrenal glands, which is why it is extremely useful in cases of jaundice or hepatitis.

7. <u>Celery, aphrodisiac properties</u>: scientists have revealed that celery is an ingredient that regulates hormones in both men and women. Some studies hypothesize that it can eliminate frigidity and even combat erectile dysfunction.

8. <u>It eliminates and prevents gallstones</u>: in the same way it works against kidney stones, it also works against gallstones in the kidney or urinary tract. By consuming celery frequently, an imminent elimination of toxins in the body can be achieved, which is essential to break down and eliminate urinary stones in the gall bladder.
9. <u>It has a crucial antibacterial action</u>: celery has many healing properties, but you should also know that its juice has enormous antibacterial powers. It has been discovered that, if taken frequently, it can help in the treatment of gastrointestinal diseases because, thanks to its antibacterial effect, it can protect the stomach mucosa from external agents that could cause damage.
10. It calms the nervous system: the juice contains an alkaline mineral, which is a component that has a calming and relaxing effect that is directly reflected in the nervous system. It is an excellent solution for all people who have suffered from an insomnia problem. For this problem, it is essential to drink at least one glass of celery juice every night, preferably one hour before going to bed.

***

Chilli pepper – Bird's-eye chilli

- Nutrient activators of sirtuin: luteolin and myricetin.

Hot pepper is a fantastic sirtuin activator and a formidable metabolism activator.

It belongs to the Solanaceae family like the potato. There are different species of chilli pepper, and the one that is most familiar to us is the classic red chilli pepper, the Cayenne one, known to be very hot.

To measure its hotness, we take a scale from 1 to 10 as the unit of measurement.

There are many varieties of chilli pepper. The known species are about 3,000.

We list some of the best known:

Poblano: (spicy 2/10) has a sweet taste, with hints of raisins. If fresh, it is known as "poblano;" while dried, it is called "ancho." In the kitchen, it is excellent paired with chestnut or grape jams and then accompanied by cheese. It is the protagonist of the Mexican sauces used to accompany the turkey.

Rocotillo: (2/10 piquancy) native of Peru, with fruity hints and a moderate spicy note; it takes on bright colors ranging from light green to red, orange to brown. It is typical of Cuban and Mexican cuisine. It gives its best in stews, sauces, vegetable soups.

Jalapeno: (spicy 2/10) typical of Mexican and Texan cuisine, it has a fragrant and not very spicy flesh. In the kitchen, it goes well with brine, vegetables, and meat.

Peter Pepper: (spiciness 3/10) fleshy and not very spicy, has unknown and ancient origins. It is not particularly fragrant, and in the kitchen, it is used just to flavor pickles, emphasize sautéed vegetables, and boiled meat.

Cayenne: (spicy 5/10) native of Mexico, it is wrongly considered the hottest chilli pepper in the world, but in reality, it is not so, because it is far surpassed by habanero chilli pepper. The long, tapered fruits lend themselves well to being dried and then preserved in powder form. It is the most widely used, not only in the Caribbean and African culture, but also in the United States and Europe.

Diavolicchio Diamante: (spiciness 5/10) is characterized by shiny fruits, elongated in shape, and a beautiful bright red color. Calabria is one of the major producers; sun-dried and ground are the protagonists on the table, and as necklaces, are hung in kitchens for winter use.

Rocoto: (spiciness 6/10) the spicy note is very marked. Widespread, especially in Peruvian cuisine to flavor meat and fish dishes, stews, and beans; or baked in the oven stuffed with meat or cheese. A hint of Rocoto is ideal to flavor honey and soya, and then accompany chicken wings or other exotic delicacies.

Habanero Chocolate: (spiciness 8/10), also known as Black Congo and native to Jamaica, is among the hottest varieties. Once ripe, the fruits go from green to dark brown. At first impact, it is incredibly spicy, but the effect disappears quickly.

Our favorite is **Thai chilli**, also known as **Bird's-eye chilli or Thai dragon**. It is a name that indicates various types of chilli peppers that are grown in Thailand and China. All Thai chilli peppers belong to the *Capsicum Annuum* species.

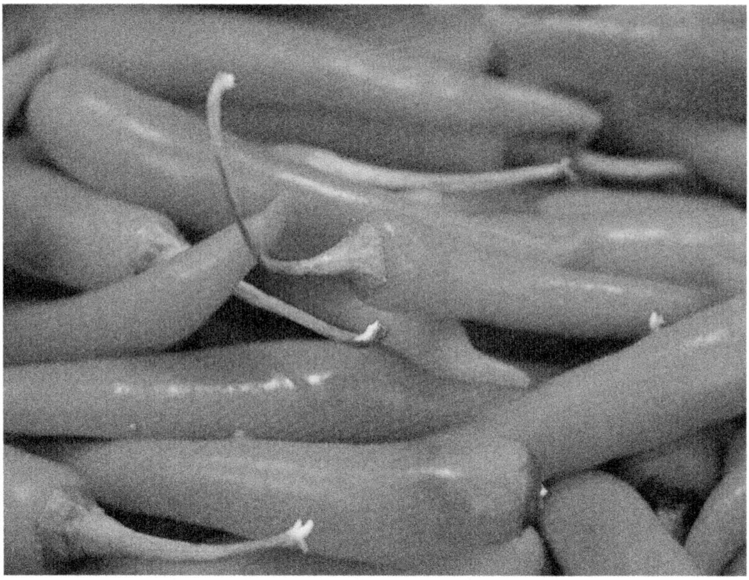

Figure 1 - Bird's-eye chilli or Thai chilli

Thai chilli peppers have an average length ranging from 5 to 10 centimeters and a width of about 2 centimeters. The fruits are green when unripe, turning a bright red and shiny skin when ripe. **The plant** grows both in height and width. We are talking about 70-100 cm. The various stems may need support. The flowers of the Thai chilli are white.

Thai chilli has a medium-high spiciness (spiciness 5/10 to 8/10). You can use Thai chilli in the kitchen to enrich practically any dish. It is ideal to use it fresh because of the exquisite sweet taste it offers.

Thai chilli is suitable for making sauces, hot oils, jams, or to be used chopped into food.

It is grown in pots or the garden.

The best time to grow Thai chilli is between July and October.

If you choose to grow it in a pot, you will need to find one with a diameter of at least 30 centimeters, and as deep. It withstands temperature drops quite well, but never below 12°C. However, it needs long exposures in full sun and germinates in about eight days when temperatures are between 25°C and 28°C.

It needs soil rich in organic matter and fresh, which is well-drained. It also requires a fertilizer with a high potassium content. It has a high water need. The seed of the seedling is easier to find on the market so that you can start with it. If, on the other hand, you want to avoid all this, go to specialist shops to buy the seedling.

If you start from the seed, you have to sow the seed at home or in a heated greenhouse. This way, you can begin as early as February. If you want to grow them outside, wait until April.

However, you can only do the transplanting when the temperatures are above 18°C, around May. The seedlings must reach a height of 10 cm.

The best way to store Thai chilli peppers is by drying them.

How to dry the Thai chilli pepper?

Thanks to its conformation, with the pulp concentrated mainly outside, this chilli pepper is easy to dry even though it is excellent eaten fresh.

If you want to eat freshly picked Thai chilli peppers, know that you can keep them in the refrigerator even for a whole week.

If you have a lot of chilli peppers, you need to find a more durable method of preservation, so you can dry them by exposing them to the sun.

Place the hot peppers on aluminum trays to speed up the process. In this way, only chilli peppers that are free of mold should be stored.

Otherwise, you can dry them in the fan dryer, in the oven, or you can store the Thai chilli peppers in oils or hot sauces.

***

Curly kale

- Sirtuin activator nutrients: kaempferol and quercetin.

Cabbage boasts enormous amounts of quercetin and kaempferol, making it a key ingredient in every diet, including the Sirt.

It is also an indigenous vegetable; ubiquitous and easy to find, as well as being cheap.

Cabbage is one of the most nutritious and healthy vegetables in the world. It should be considered fundamental for our diet, because of the richness and variety of its beneficial properties.

In the cabbage family, we find curly kale, black and red cabbage, savoy cabbage, head cabbage, broccoli, and cauliflower.

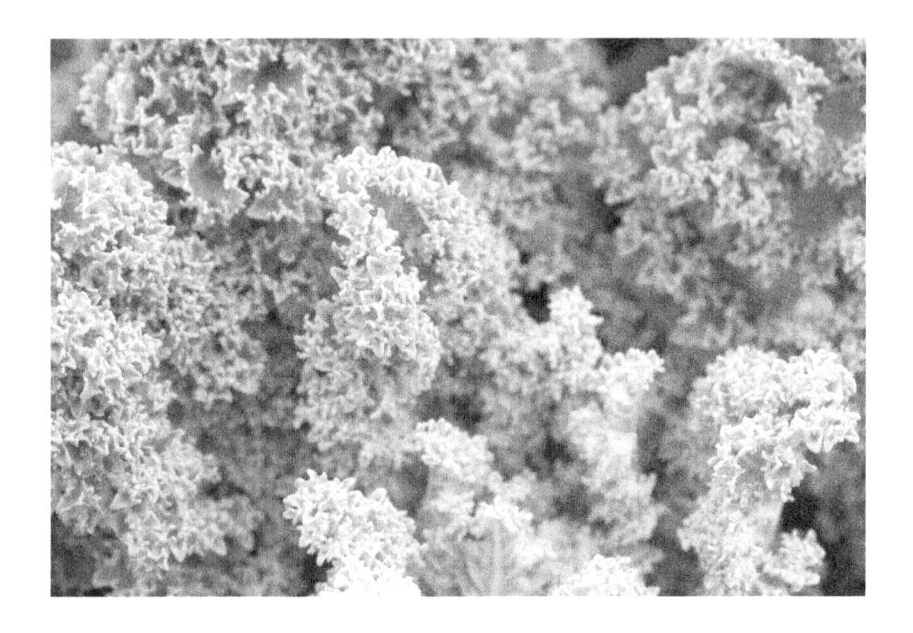

1. Natural anti-inflammatory

Among the beneficial characteristics of cabbage are its anti-inflammatory properties. Inflammation is the leading cause of diseases such as arthritis, heart disease, and autoimmune diseases, which can appear due to excessive consumption of animal products. Cabbage is a potent natural anti-inflammatory that can prevent and relieve inflammatory diseases.

2. Richer in iron than meat

Cabbage. It contains more iron per calorie than steak. The assimilation of iron contained in foods of vegetable origin is facilitated by the consumption of foods rich in vitamin C. Also, this vegetable has more calcium per calorie than milk. Our body would be able to assimilate vegetable calcium even better than calcium from dairy products.

3. Rich in fiber

Fiber is a macronutrient that we need to take every day. A lack of fiber in the diet can cause digestive and cardiac problems and even lead to the appearance of tumors. Foods that are very rich in protein, such as meat, do not contain fiber. A regular portion of cabbage provides our body with 5% of the fiber we need every day, along with 2 grams of protein.

4. Rich in fatty acids (omega-3 and omega-6)

Omega-3 fatty acids play an essential role in maintaining health. A portion of cabbage contains about 120 milligrams of omega-3 fatty acids and about 92 milligrams of omega-6 fatty acids. The essential fatty acids must be taken every day. Other food sources that contain them are nuts, oil, and linseed.

5. Rich in calcium

Cabbage is one of the significant vegetable sources of calcium: 3/4 cups of kale contain as much calcium as a cup of cow's milk. Raw green cabbage, for example, contains 72 mg of calcium per 100 gr.

6. Strengthens the immune system

Cabbage is a valuable source of beneficial substances that help the immune system to defend our body against diseases and attacks by germs and bacteria.

7. Natural antioxidant against free radicals

It is rich in vitamin A and vitamin C, but also in carotenoids and flavonoids with strong antioxidant properties, which with their activities, contribute to the prevention of illnesses and premature aging. Cabbages contain over 45 types of flavonoids, with quercitin in the first place. The flavonoids present in cabbage combine antioxidant and anti-inflammatory benefits, making it a suitable food for the prevention of oxidative stress.

8. Detoxifying and Antitumoral

It has been scientifically proven that the consumption of cabbage is effective in reducing the risk of contracting certain types of cancer, with particular reference to breast, bladder, ovarian, colon, and prostate cancer. Cabbage consumption helps our body to detoxify. Some of the components present in cabbage would be able to regulate the elimination of toxins at a genetic level.

9. Lowers blood pressure

Cabbage is an excellent ally against hypertension and high blood pressure thanks to the presence of glutamic acid, an amino acid which, as has been demonstrated, contributes significantly to lowering blood pressure.

10. Protects heart and arteries

Recent research says that these vegetables, thanks to the sulforaphane contained in them, can reactivate Nrf2. This protein is responsible for keeping blood vessels free of fat, which is the main cause of cardiovascular diseases such as angina, heart attack, stroke, and, indeed, arteriosclerosis.

As nutritious as meat, but more sustainable

Not to be underestimated is the aspect of sustainability. We are now well aware of the environmental impact of intensive livestock farming on the planet. You only need to make a quick comparison to know that it only takes 60 days to taste fresh cabbages after sowing, while cattle breeding will take 18 to 24 months before new meat is available. Cabbages are very resistant, even in cold climates, and can quickly be grown on farms or in the vegetable garden, with less water and energy consumption than is necessary to keep cattle reared for slaughter.

How to enjoy the benefits

Steaming allows the cabbage to maintain the necessary nutrients to lower cholesterol. Steam does not alter the quality of the vegetable fibers present in the cabbage too much.

***

Cocoa

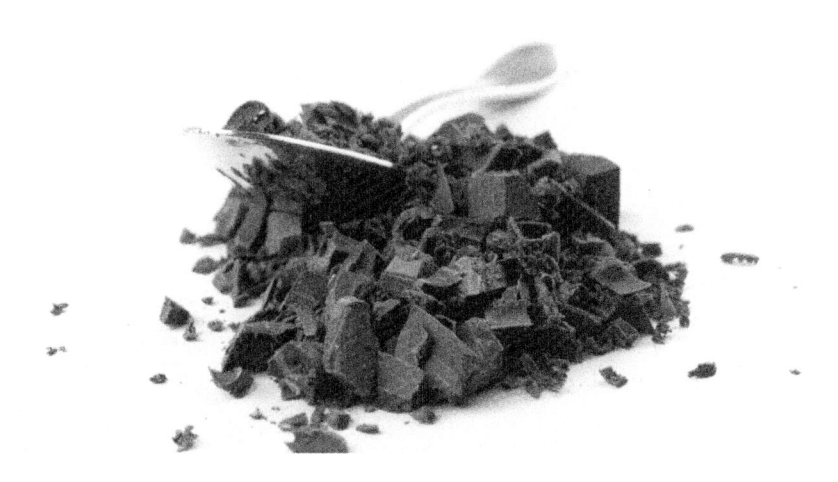

- Sirtuin Activating Nutrients: Epicatechin

To be considered a real sirtfood, chocolate must be dark and contain at least 85% solid cocoa.

Chocolate is often treated with alkalizing agents to reduce acidity and give it a darker color. This treatment is known as the "Dutch method" and it drastically reduces the flavonoid activator content of sirtuin, thus compromising the health properties of the product.

Here are all the benefits of dark chocolate

1. Dark chocolate is antidepressant
Having clarified the origins and the name of this delicacy, let's see what the main properties of dark chocolate are. If you feel

down, eat a piece of chocolate, taste it slowly, and you'll feel better right away. Chocolate stimulates the secretion of endorphins, the hormones of happiness that can give you a pleasant feeling of well-being almost immediately. And that's not all. Dark chocolate can be considered a natural antidepressant, because it increases the production of serotonin, an excitatory neurotransmitter that otherwise causes a pathological lowering of mood.

2. *Protects the skin*

It was always believed that chocolate was responsible for pimples and acne problems. In truth, the most recent research has reduced the accusations made against chocolate, considering other foods such as milk and its derivatives, cakes, sweets, and sugars in general, as more responsible. Chocolate, on the contrary, thanks to its antioxidant properties, can protect the skin from the harmful effects of UV rays and keep the skin hydrated.

3. *Fights muscle cramps*

If you suffer from muscle cramps, you probably have a deficiency of magnesium, the essential mineral for the body, because it ensures the proper functioning of the cells, fights muscle pain, and the appearance of annoying cramps. Magnesium can be found in quantities in foods such as figs, dates, dried fruit, soy sprouts, and of course, also in bitter cocoa. For this reason, dark chocolate is often consumed by sportsmen and women who suffer from cramps and muscle pain.

4. Ideal for those who suffer from anemia

Dark chocolate has about 2 mg of iron for every 100 grams. For this reason, it is particularly recommended for those who suffer from anemia or women with a very abundant menstrual flow.

5. Chocolate is good for the heart

Dark chocolate is good for the heart, increasing the concentration of antioxidants in the blood by 20%. But be careful: this benefit is only linked to dark chocolate. Milk chocolate has no beneficial effect on the blood and heart! Dark chocolate contains a very high amount of polyphenols (specifical flavonoids). These substances can fight cholesterol, lower blood pressure, regulate vascular tone, and the degree of restriction of the blood vessel lumen. Real prevention for cardiovascular diseases such as stroke and heart attack.

6. Good mood ally

I mean, as you may have guessed, chocolate is a real ally of good humor and health. Eating chocolate promotes the production of serotonin, which can help you against sadness or bad mood. So here's my advice: always keep a bar of chocolate with you, it can help you straighten out a bad day.

7. Chocolate is also an antioxidant

Don't forget the antioxidant effect of dark chocolate and cocoa: they even seem to have an antioxidant power superior even to that of fruit. Finally, did you know that chocolate is rich in minerals? Iron, magnesium, calcium, and potassium are just some of those present in 50 grams of dark chocolate. Now you have no excuse to resist!

Who's not good with chocolate?

Be careful, though, because dark chocolate is not suitable for everyone. It increases blood sugar levels, and for this reason, it is not recommended for people who have diabetes: it is better to reduce its consumption or avoid it totally when blood sugar levels are already high. If, on the contrary, blood sugar levels are under control, two squares of chocolate are certainly not bad. Dark chocolate improves mood, lowers blood pressure, reduces cardiovascular risk, and seems to improve sugar metabolism.

***

Coffee

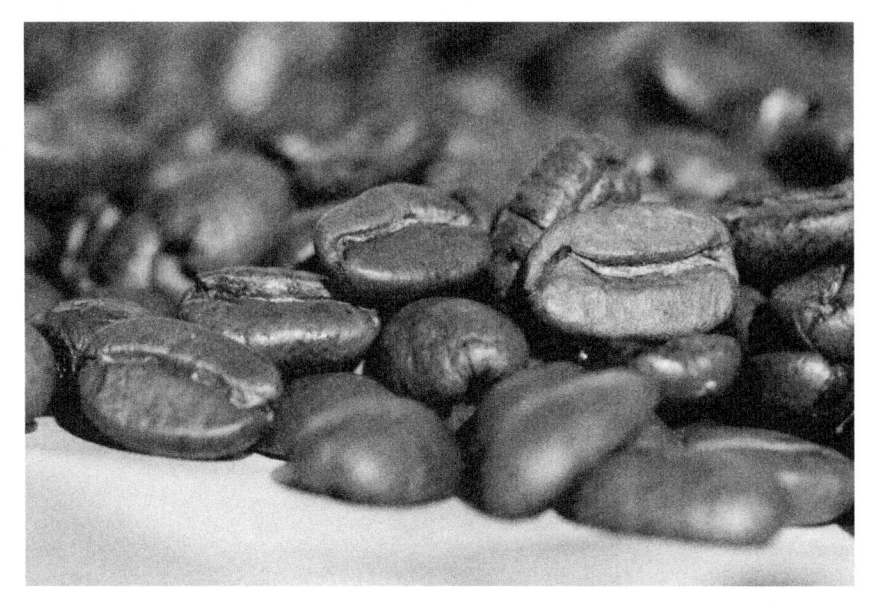

- Activating nutrients of sirtuin: caffeic acid and chlorogenic acid.

Coffee is a real treasure trove of plant compounds with great health benefits. Coffee drinkers have a significantly lower risk of developing certain types of cancer, neurodegenerative diseases, and even diabetes.

It also protects the liver and helps to keep it healthy.

1. Improved concentration and energy

Thanks to the effect of the active ingredient of coffee known as caffeine, this drink can make us feel more energetic, helping us to wake up better and concentrate more, because caffeine is a stimulating substance that acts directly on our brain.

2. *It helps burn excess fat*

Always the caffeine contained in coffee can improve our metabolism by about 11%, forcing our body to burn a greater amount of calories, thus promoting slimming. It should certainly come as no surprise: caffeine has been used as an ingredient for years in the field of weight loss supplements, such as thermogenesis.

3. *Protects against cardiovascular diseases*

We are often mistakenly led to think that coffee increases blood pressure leading to problems. In reality, the increase is so small and not very persistent that this statement can be considered untrue.

4. *It contains a vast source of antioxidants*

Drinking coffee allows us to take a considerable amount of antioxidants that we know help to protect against free radicals, one of the major causes of cellular damage.

5. *Protects the liver*

The liver is a vital organ for our body that performs an incredible number of functions. Coffee acts as real protection for our liver.

***

Extra virgin olive oil

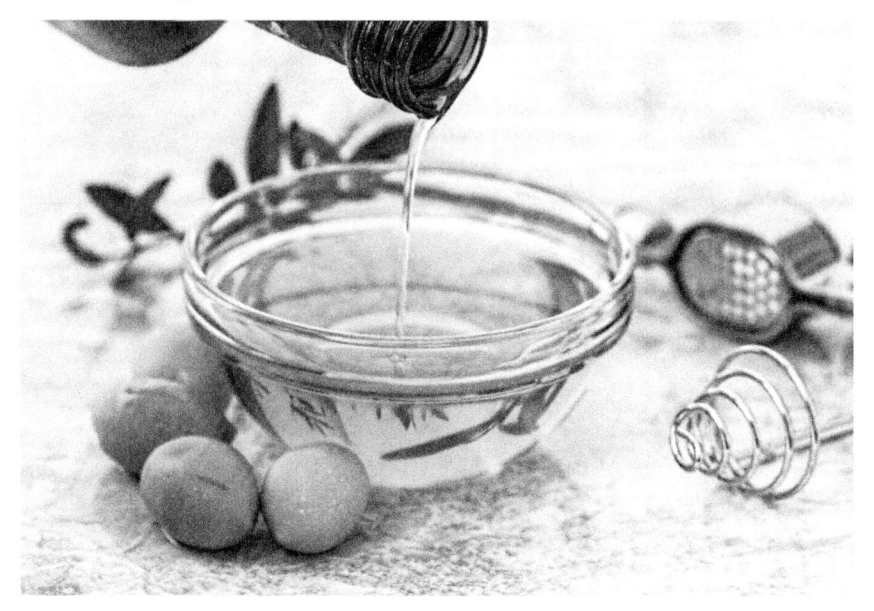

- Sirtuin activator nutrients: oleuropein and hydroxytyrosol.

Hippocrates already mentioned olive oil as "the cure for all ills," about 2000 years before modern science showed its excellent benefits.

When it comes to olive oil, it is essential to buy extra virgin olive oil.

Virgin oil is obtained only through the mechanical pressing of fruits and in conditions that do not lead to the deterioration of the oil. In this way, you can be sure of the quality of the product and its polyphenol content.

"Extra virgin' refers to the first pressing of the fruit ('virgin' refers to the second pressing), which gives a product of better quality and taste.

The use of extra virgin olive oil is very ancient: the roots of its history can be found in the Middle East and, in particular, in Palestine. Here, has been found some of the oldest oil mills ever existed, and dated several millennia before Christ. From Palestine, this critical food was brought to Egypt, Greece, and throughout the Mediterranean: it was introduced in Italy by the Greeks, followed by the Etruscans. The Etruscans gave it its current name, "oil," which derives from the word *eleiva*.

Extra virgin olive oil is among the best fats you can choose to use in your daily diet, even when you are on a diet.

Benefits:

1. It lowers cholesterol and protects your heart.

The lipids of which the oil is composed are 75% oleic acid; then linoleic acid and palmitic acid. These are monounsaturated fats that make extra virgin olive oil a valuable ally of your cardiovascular system.

So-called "good" fatty acids help your heart because they keep bad cholesterol (LDL) under control and enhance 'good' cholesterol (HDL), which cleans the arteries. Phytosterols are plant substances that can hinder the intestinal absorption of cholesterol and reduce LDL cholesterol found in the blood. Thanks to them, the fatty acids in extra virgin olive oil have a fully effective preventive action against cardiovascular diseases, including heart attacks, thus protecting your heart.

2. It slows down cellular aging.

Extra virgin olive oil has a fundamental antioxidant function, thanks above all to vitamin E and many polyphenols. These two nutrients together perform an exceptional part of contrasting free radicals, the cause of cellular aging.

3. Extra virgin olive oil is excellent for obtaining elastic skin.

Extra virgin olive oil is a natural source of vitamin E, considered the vitamin of beauty because it is a powerful antioxidant that protects cell membranes from aging processes.

With one tablespoon of extra virgin olive oil a day, you will take 15% of the recommended daily dose of vitamin E, thus ensuring a preventive action against tumor and degenerative diseases, and protecting DNA and cell membranes from damage caused by free radicals.

Also, thanks to the support of carotenoids and vitamin A, which promote collagen synthesis and the formation of new cells; it allows you to have elastic, strong, and healthy skin.

4. It strengthens your immune system and helps you in times of stress.

This mix of substances beneficial for your body and acting in synergy, also has the effect of strengthening your immune system. Extra virgin olive oil is also indicated in periods of particular fatigue:

- stress
- seasons changes
- examination period

- special events
- childbirth
- pollution
- anxiety

because the vitamins and mineral salts, make it a valuable remedy.

5. Extra virgin olive oil is a support for the diet.

Extra virgin olive oil, with 99% lipids, is certainly caloric: for every 100 grams, there are 900 calories. However, this is not a good reason to remove it from your diet if you are on a diet. When you consume extra virgin olive oil, the intake of fat-soluble vitamins, such as A, D, E, and K, is facilitated, and so olive oil remains the best seasoning, even with its caloric intake.

Without this good fat, some vitamins taken with fruits and vegetables are lost and like a part of calcium, which depends precisely on a fat-soluble vitamin D to be absorbed in the best way.

The extra virgin olive oil, thanks to its fats, promotes the sense of satiety, and protects the stomach from inflammation, improving digestion and avoiding abdominal swelling linked to the lazy intestine.

***

Lovage

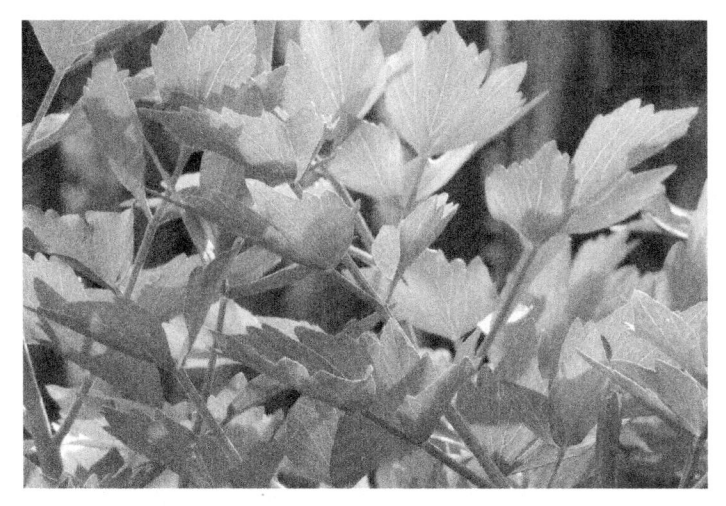

- Nutrient activators of sirtuin: quercitin.

Lovage is an extremely versatile plant, with a celery and parsley flavor, but much more durable.

It was considered an aphrodisiac, so much so that even Charlemagne ordered it to be planted in his garden (it was called "parsley of love").

Unfortunately, today, we are no longer used to its taste, but its beneficial properties are undeniable.

The lovage, *Levisticum officinalis*, is a plant belonging to the botanical family Apiaceae or Umbelliferae.

It is a close relative of leaf celery and celeriac, as well as other plants of the same family, such as fennel, parsley, carrots, dill, chervil, and green anise.

The species is native to Persia, the present Iran, and in ancient times has started to spread in central and southern Europe. It is often encountered spontaneously in the pre-Alpine and Apennine zones, from 500 to 1.500 m of altitude.

Its preferred habitat is uncultivated meadows, both in half shade and in full sun; the important thing is that it has a humid and well-drained soil.

The lovage plant.

Lovage is a perennial herbaceous plant. An excellent rusticity and high vigor characterize it since it can exceed 2 m in height.

The plant stands with long hollow-sectioned stems and a rounded shape, which branch upwards. The single stem is green, but with reddish shades.

The lovage has a large taproot from which numerous lateral roots branch out. These can descend to a depth of up to 40 cm. The leaves of the lovage are large, inserted alternately on the stem, and carried by a long, hollow petiole. They are engraved, toothed, and deep green in color; when young, they resemble those of the common celery.

This plant flowers from June and throughout the summer, while in autumn, the lovage seeds become ripen, elongated and flattened small achenes. The weight of 1000 seeds does not exceed 10 g.

Lovage cultivation.

Growing lovage is a rather straightforward practice, as it is a rustic and, therefore, very resistant plant. Because of its pungent taste, it is often preferred to common celery as an aromatic plant, and is perfect for cultivation in mountain areas.

Remember that mountain celery is a perennial plant, and therefore needs a space in the garden where it can grow undisturbed. For example, it could be profitable to place a plant of *Levisticum officinalis* next to sage or rosemary, which are other common perennial aromatic plants that we encounter in our gardens.

It withstands harsh winter temperatures well, so it doesn't need protection from frost. On the contrary, if we are growing it in regions with sweltering summers, it is better to place it in half shade or use a shading net to prevent the leaves from yellowing.

The lovage grows well in loose, deep, and fresh agricultural land, with a good supply of organic matter. On the other hand, it escapes those that are too clayey and asphyxiated, which give rise to water stagnation.

The properties of lovage

Lovage is known for its medicinal properties, given the significant presence of active ingredients. It contains resins, tannins, sugars, vitamin C, pectins, acids, and essential oils.

The use of mountain celery was widespread in the monastic workshop and appreciated for its properties:

- diuretics
- antiemetics
- anti-rheumatic
- deodorants
- antiseptic
- carminative
- tonics
- digestive

It was used not only as fresh food to season dishes but also in the form of infusions and decoctions. The dry rhizomatous root, on the other hand, is boiled and is an excellent adjuvant to the regular activity of the kidneys.

Lovage in the kitchen

Lovage leaves have always been appreciated in the kitchen for their intense aroma and spicy and persistent taste.

It was the aromatic plant par excellence of the ancient Romans, who used it as we consume parsley and common celery today. This mountain celery can give a pleasant taste to salads, soups, and meats. This plant is used as an essential component of the vegetable nuts, with which the broth is prepared. The sprouts are eaten alone and are delicious when seasoned with extra-virgin olive oil and balsamic vinegar.

***

Matcha Green Tea

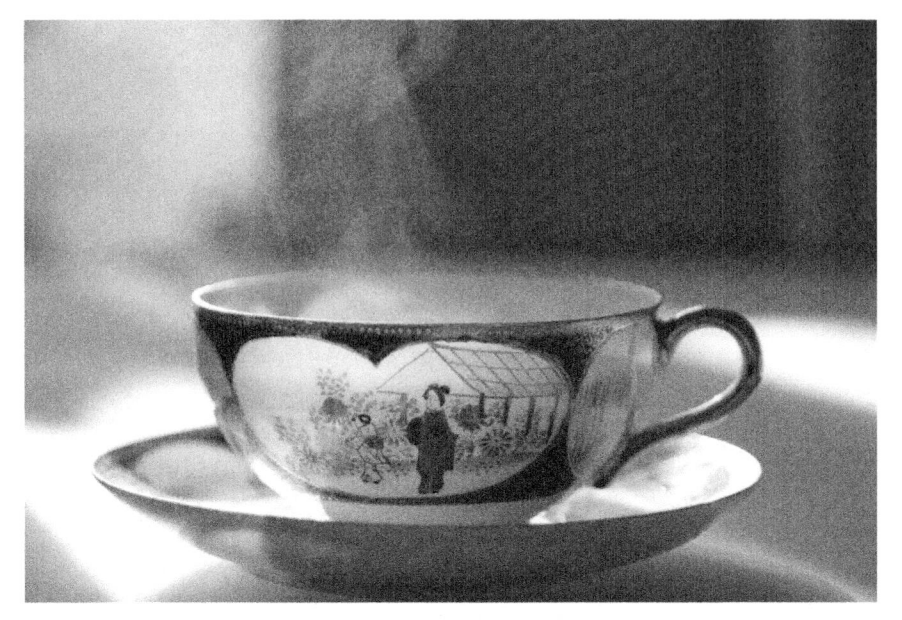

- Sirtuin activator nutrients: epigallocatechin gallate (EGCG).

Matcha tea grows in 90% shade, while ordinary green tea grows in direct sunlight.

The matcha leaves are crushed into a powder using a stone. Unlike green tea, which is infused and then drunk, this powder dissolves in water and is ingested.

The advantage of this method is that it allows the intake of a more considerable amount of EGCG, a substance that activates sirtuin.

The matcha tea is the king of green teas that would contain 137 times more antioxidants than traditional green tea. Matcha tea, or Japanese green tea, has superior antioxidant properties compared to any other green tea. Recent studies have shown that matcha tea leaves contain 137 times the antioxidant content of regular green tea, as well as polyphenols, and several amino acids, which reduce physical and psychological stress, and glutamic acid that acts on the central nervous system.

Matcha tea is a variety of green tea that Japanese growers grow under the sun and whose leaves are harvested by hand and then turned into powder through the use of stone mills. Thanks to this processing, matcha tea is very precious and excellent powder with an intense emerald green color, and particularly rich in vitamins, mineral salts, chlorophyll, and carotene.

Health benefits

This powder is obtained from the best quality leaves of Gyokuro, crumbled in singular crushers. The way matcha tea is prepared gives it a higher concentration of substances than the usual infusion. In particular, matcha tea is rich in vitamins B1, B2, and C, beta-carotene, mineral salts, polyphenols, and caffeine, which promotes a state of vigilance.

Skin. Matcha tea is synonymous with antioxidants: Matcha contains 70 mg per gram of catechins, a much higher amount than that provided in green tea bags. It is, therefore, an excellent anti-aging, draining, and detoxifying remedy. Not only that, matcha tea also proves to be a remedy for preventing sunburn and protecting our skin from possible damage caused by ultraviolet rays. Its protective action would be due to the high content of polyphenols present in the leaves from which the powder is obtained.

Digestion. It calms the mucous membranes of the stomach and intestine and is useful in the treatment of diseases of nervous or inflammatory origin that affect the digestive system. Also, it is an effective remedy against gastric hyperacidity and protects the liver.

Slimming diets. Matcha tea can reduce the feeling of hunger so that it can be used in low-calorie foods, also thanks to its diuretic effect that helps in weight loss.

Finally, matcha would be able to prevent heart attacks or stroke, keep diabetes and hypertension at bay, and reduce blood cholesterol levels.

Contraindications

Of course, not even matcha tea can be abused. Tea contains a lot of caffeine and polyphenols, and drinking too much or too concentrated could cause tremors and palpitations or indigestion. Also, make sure that the tea does not interfere with medicines or supplements you are already taking. Some components of tea may interact with certain substances.

Where is it found?

The best matcha, only powdered and of the highest quality, comes from the Uji Tawara region, which seems to have the optimum soil and climatic conditions for tea growing. You can find it in herbal shops, natural food stores, or easily online.

Choose the organic matcha grade 1 for which only the first sprouts are used, while in the cheaper matcha (grade 2 and above), you can also mix second and third harvest leaves.

***

Medjool dates

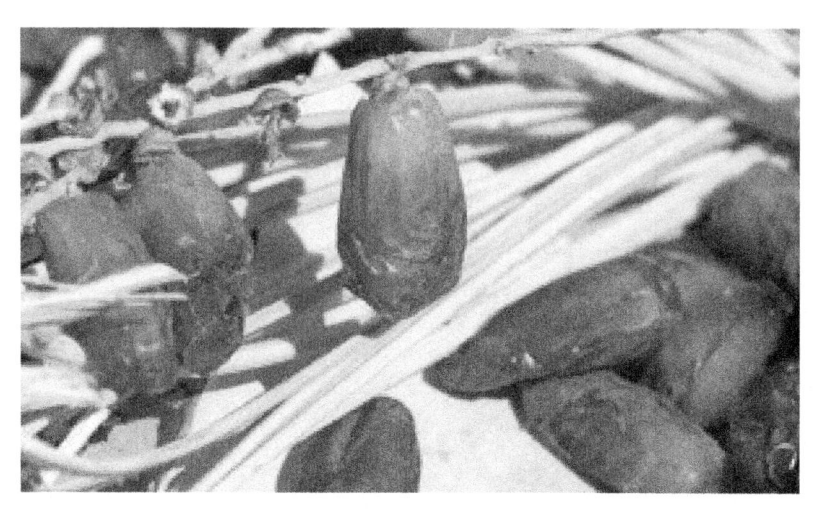

- Sirtuin activating nutrients: Gallic acid and caffeic acid.

The inclusion in this list of Medjool dates can be extraordinary at first because they are composed of 66% sugar.

This substance is not related to the production of sirtuin and should be consumed in small quantities.

However, the sugar present in dates is very different from refined sugar and is balanced by polyphenols that activate the production of sirtuin.

These dates are also allies in combating the risk of diabetes and heart disease.

The "Medjoul" date, also known as "jumbo" date due to its size, is an Israeli variety characterized by a rather dark color, with creamy pulp and high sugar content, as well as a tiny kernel. The

"Medjoul" dates are the most prized, and available all year round; thanks to their excellent preservation capacity.

Dates do not contain cholesterol and have a low-fat content. They are a source of energy immediately available to the body due to their sugar content. They are a good source of potassium, while at the same time being low in sodium.

***

Parsley

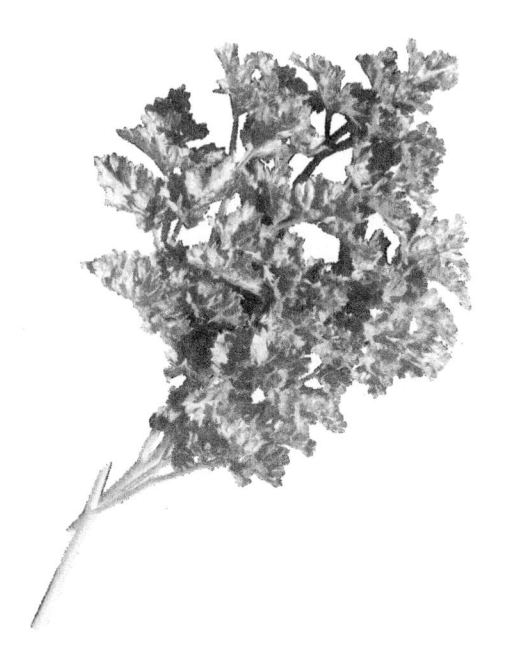

- Sirtuin activator nutrients: apigenin and myricetin.

Too often in the kitchen, we tend to use a small sprig of parsley only for decorative purposes.

This plant is an excellent source of apigenin, a nutrient that activates the production of sirtuin and is rarely found in such significant quantities in other foods.

Parsley is a spice rich in vitamins and minerals, which protects bones and hair and has a diuretic and pressure regulating action.

Parsley (*Petroselinum sativum*) is a biennial herbaceous plant that belongs to the Apiaceae family, having a robust yellowish-white taproot and fleshy. The leaves are long petiolate, rosette-shaped, dark green in color, wholly glabrous and have a jagged triangular outline. The inflorescence is an umbrella formed by about fifty small flowers with five white petals that are sometimes yellow-greenish, and which produce small oval, flattened, grey-brown seeds. Properties and benefits of parsley abound in the kitchen and in the daily diet. Parsley should preferably be used raw to preserve all the features of its leaves. It is an aromatic herb with many therapeutic and curative properties, given its high content of vitamins and mineral salts, which deteriorate with the heat of cooking. A spoonful of chopped parsley leaves contains the same amount of vitamin C as a small orange (two-thirds of the daily requirement). Vitamin C strengthens the immune system, strengthens the circulatory system, and fluidifies the blood. Parsley is also an excellent source of beta-carotene, with an antioxidant action for the skin; calcium is fundamental for remineralizing bones and helps to keep hair and nails healthy. The roots are rich in potassium, which gives the plant diuretic and pressure regulating properties. However, its use should not be excessive or in large quantities for pregnant women.

Parsley in the kitchen is among the most widely used aromatic herbs. It should always be added at the end of cooking so as not to compromise the essential oil, which gives fragrance and flavor. It goes well with many foods of the Mediterranean diet, mainly when used in gravies to season barbecued and marinated meat.

Because of its particularity of being used practically everywhere, parsley was the inspiration for the famous saying: "be everywhere like parsley." Oshawa, the father of macrobiotics, says that "a bowl of chopped raw parsley should never be missing on our table!" It seems that it was already known in ancient times, and the Greeks used it not as an aroma, but as a decoration for tombs, flowerbeds, and mainly for its therapeutic powers on the disorders of kidneys, bladder, and toothache. The Romans, however, used it primarily in the kitchen, and to make garlands for banquet guests. The Romans' neighbors, the Etruscans, considered parsley a plant with magical properties, and for this reason, they made miraculous ointments out of it.

***

Red chicory

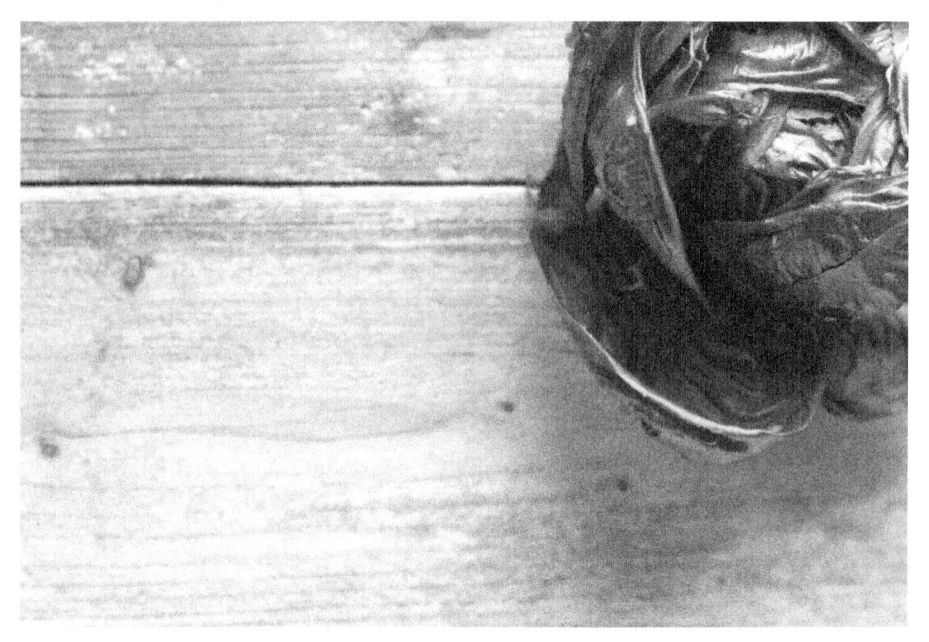

- Nutrient activators of sirtuin: luteolin.

Red chicory (also known as radicchio) can be more challenging to find. Alternatively, you can use yellow chicory. Its sour taste adds a special note to an extra virgin olive oil-based condiment.
Loved by many for its particular bitterish taste, the red chicory belongs to the chicory family. Whether eaten raw or cooked, it lends itself well to enrich many recipes, but it also has many useful properties for our organism.

What it contains:

- Very few calories: its weight is composed of about 94-96% water.
- Mineral salts in quantity, in particular potassium, iron, calcium, and phosphorus.
- Vitamins: it boasts Vitamins of group B, Vitamin C, and Vitamin K.
- Fibers: in high quantity.
- Polyphenols: with antioxidant properties.

The presence within it of all these precious substances translates into several benefits for those who regularly consume red chicory. The most important of these are given by:

1. The ANTIOXIDANT properties. The particular mix of vitamins and polyphenols gives this food useful antioxidant properties, which help to prevent aging diseases and keep the body young and healthy.

2. DISINTOSSICANT properties. With antioxidant properties of red chicory in their role of tissue renewal, there are also purifying properties. The bitter substances contained within it, also exert a stimulus to the activity of the liver and the purification of the body from waste substances.

3. DIGESTIVE properties. The same bitter substances are also useful to stimulate the production of gastric juices and therefore favor better and faster digestion at the stomach level.

4. The LASSATIVE properties. The high fiber content makes red chicory a beneficial vegetable in fighting constipation.

5. The health of the CARDIOVASCULAR system. It contains anthocyanins, a particular type of polyphenols, which, thanks to their anti-inflammatory and antioxidant properties, help to keep blood vessels healthy, thus reducing the risk of developing disorders in the cardiovascular system.

Because of its particular taste, red chicory is generally not eaten alone but accompanied by other sweeter foods that soften the bitterness a bit.

While raw radicchio is excellent with red beetroot or carrots, when cooked, it goes very well with vegetables such as pumpkin or potato, as well as being an excellent condiment for first or second courses such as risottos, savory pies, and meat dishes.

***

Red Onion

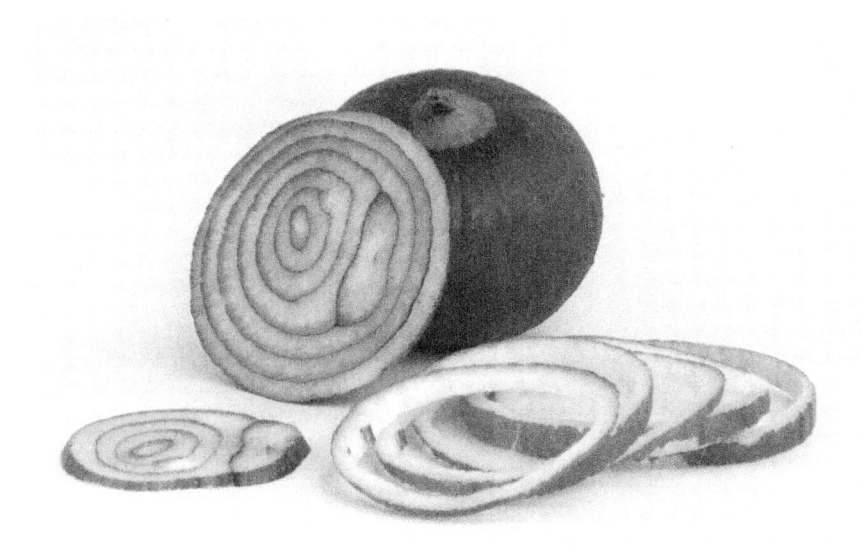

- Nutrient activators of sirtuin: quercitin.

Red onion has the highest concentration of quercetin, but yellow onions also contain significant amounts. It is essential to eat them raw, to keep the nutrient levels unchanged: fried onions lose 20% of quercitin during the process, a percentage that reaches 65% if cooked in the microwave, and 75% if boiled.
Red onions have a particular and unique ovoid or slightly roundish shape, red-purple wrapping, and white inner tunics. The taste is sweet, highly digestible. Called also *Tropea onions*, they are very suitable in the diets of heart patients for their anti-sclerotic power. For the high content of vitamins and iron, they are indicated to combat states of the physical deficit.

The very high content of flavonoids, phenols, quercetin, and mineral salts, in combination with other purifying minerals, contained in these purple onions considerably reduce the risk of cancer of the larynx, liver, colon, and ovaries.

Due to their richness in chromium sulfates, Tropea onions are useful in the treatment of diabetes (they have the power to reduce blood sugar). They also prevent arterial hypertension, atherosclerosis, and other cardiovascular diseases as they intervene in the regulation of triglycerides and blood cholesterol levels (fats that reduce the lumen of the arteries).

A good onion must be firm, without mold and sprouts. It is crucial to use no refrigerator to store onions. They should be stored in a cool, dry place at room temperature. If you can keep them at the right temperature, they can stay for 2 or 3 weeks.

The red onion can enrich, with its taste, many dishes and can be eaten raw in tasty salads or cooked as a base for soups. This particular variety, known as Tropea red onion, can be used as a base for jams to accompany cheese; pickled onions or tasty onion tarts can be prepared with bulbs.

***

Red wine

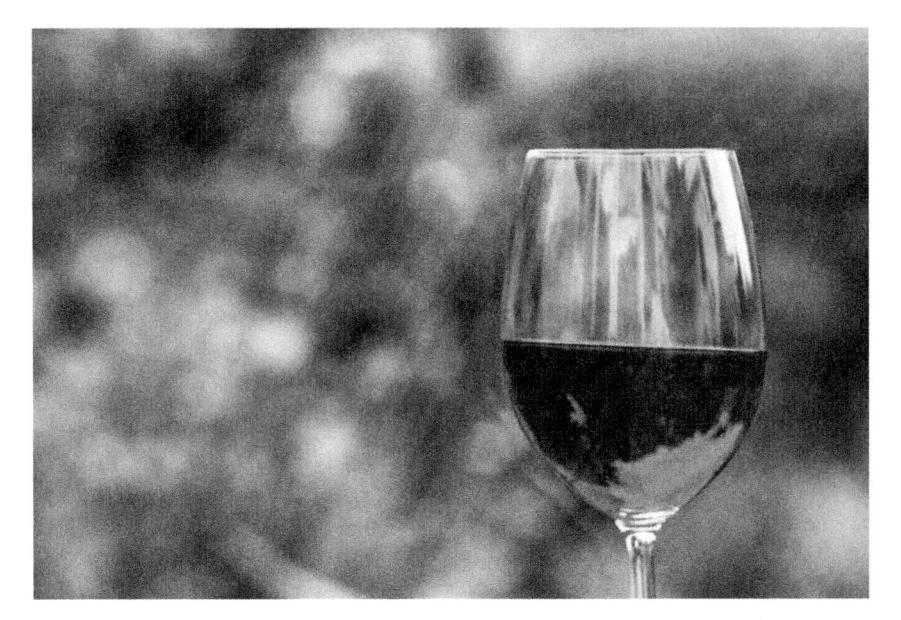

- Sirtuin activator nutrients: resveratrol and piceatannol.

Red wine is the original sirtfood, with which the base of research of this diet started and which has unleashed all the frenzy born around these foods.

Its resveratrol content, along with another input activator of sirtuin, piceatannol, is considered one of the critical reasons for the length of life and slender figures associated with the traditional French lifestyle.

The wine that contains more resveratrol than all the others is Pinot Noir.

When talking about the benefits associated with the consumption of red wine, the first molecule that comes to mind is, therefore, resveratrol (on which there are dozens and dozens of approved scientific studies). This phenol is attributed to metabolic properties such as antioxidant, antibacterial, antifungal, anti-tumor, anti-inflammatory, and blood thinning.

Under certain conditions, a glass of red wine a day may reduce the incidence of clot-related stroke by up to 50%. Resveratrol also seems to protect the brain from cognitive decline related to Alzheimer's disease.

Recently, in analyzing the composition of red wine, scientists at the "University of California at Davis"[1] discovered another group of molecules capable of fighting excess cholesterol in the blood. These are saponins, which are alcohol-soluble foaming substances, capable of binding cholesterol in the intestine (including in bile salts) and reducing its absorption.

Research by the Oregon State's College of Agricultural Studies[2], on the other hand, has observed the reaction of guinea pigs to a nutritional regime rich in fat, with and without red wine extracts. All mice showed the same metabolic consequences as overweight, sedentary humans, but those fed red wine extract revealed lower fat accumulation in the liver and lower glycemic levels. The molecule responsible for this reaction would be ellagic acid (also present in many vegetables and fruits, such as pomegranate), which is a phenolic antioxidant able to hinder the

___

[1] https://www.ucdavis.edu/news/genomics-breakthrough-paves-way-climate-tolerant-wine-grape-varieties
[2] https://owri.oregonstate.edu/

accumulation of fat in cells and oppose the development of new adipocytes.

As if that were not enough, red wine is also rich in quercetin. This flavonoid is a metabolic inhibitor of certain enzymes involved in the inflammatory response. The antioxidant functions of quercetin are to restore tocopherols (Vit. E), detoxify cells from superoxide, and decrease nitric oxide secretion during inflammation. Also, according to the American Cancer Society, this flavonoid acts as a powerful anti-tumor, especially at the colon level.

Red wine is rich in so-called tannins. These phenolic compounds, responsible for the red pigment, are very famous for their potential beneficial action at the cardiovascular level.

***

Rocket Salad

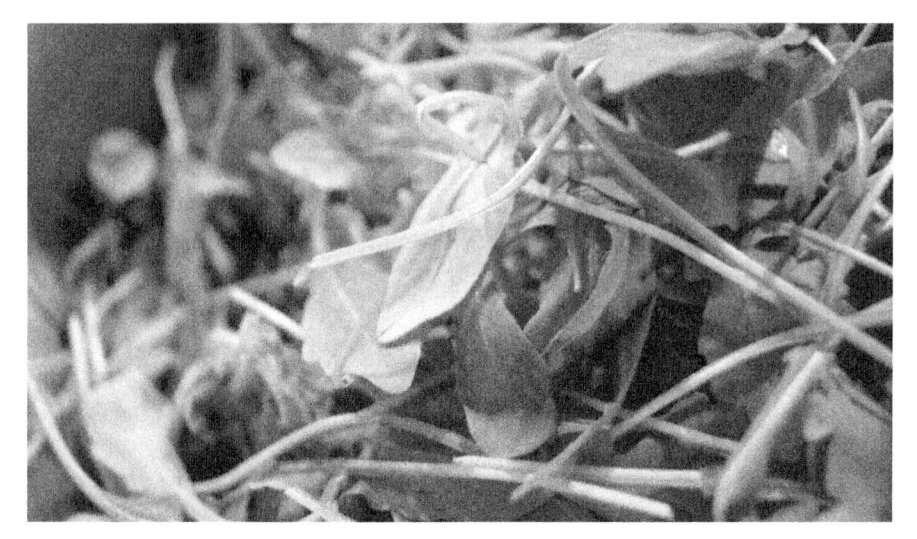

- Sirtuin activator nutrients: quercetin and kaempferol.

The rocket was first cultivated in Ancient Rome, where it was considered an aphrodisiac.

Two types are widespread: salad rocket and wild rocket. Both are two excellent activators of sirtuin.

Rocket is a herbaceous plant belonging to the Brassicaceae (Cruciferae) family, the same as cabbage and broccoli. It is native to the Mediterranean area, where it grows spontaneously.

There are two types: the cultivated one, whose scientific name is Eruca Sativa, and the wild one (Diplotaxix *tenuifolia*). The plants are similar but differ in taste, color, and leaves.

The cultivated rocket is an annual plant, has a less intense taste, and has white flowers and more full, rounded leaves at the top.

The rocket salad is cultivated in spring and has a minimal life cycle, as the leaves are harvested a few weeks after sowing. Both types have numerous nutritional properties.

The rocket has few calories (25 calories per 100 g of food) that is ideal to consume during the diet; has a high content of water, minerals, and vitamins; and it is rich in antioxidants, which fight free radicals and exert a preventive action against cancer.

The rocket is rich in elements essential for the proper functioning of various cellular processes and indispensable for the protection of the body from multiple aggressions. Calcium, Magnesium, and Potassium are the most present minerals, while the most abundant vitamins are vitamin C and vitamin K together with folates. Rocket also has excellent content of antioxidants such as beta-carotene, lutein, and zeaxanthin.

Calcium: The rocket has a good calcium content, a mineral that is a fundamental constituent of bones and teeth, so its proper intake is vital for the health of the bone apparatus and the structure of teeth. Calcium is also essential for the health of the heart and muscular system. *Magnesium:* a deficiency of this mineral can lead to nervousness, insomnia, and muscle cramps. It is because magnesium is involved in processes such as the transmission of nerve impulses and muscle contraction.

Potassium: This mineral lowers blood pressure, facilitating the elimination of excess fluid and thus counteracting water retention and cellulite. It intervenes, like magnesium, in the transmission of nerve impulses and the process of muscle contraction. It is also essential to regulate heart rate and pH.

Vitamin K: It has mainly an anti-hemorrhagic function, but also protects the bone apparatus and regulates the inflammatory response.

Beta-carotene: This element protects cells from free radicals, thanks to its powerful antioxidant action. It represents the precursor of vitamin A or Retinol, which is essential for proper visual function and intervenes in the processes of cell growth and repair; Lutein and zeaxanthin: present in the retina, these two antioxidants protect the eyes from the harmful effects of light radiation.

The consumption of the rocket offers several health benefits. Let us now go into this aspect, analyzing in detail all the properties of this food.

✓ It is remineralizing. Thanks to its essential mineral salt content; arugula consumption is ideal for replenishing salts lost through summer sweating or after physical activity. Unlike other green leafy vegetables, the rocket does not contain many oxalates, which hinder the absorption of minerals.

✓ It has a digestive function. Rocket has digestive properties as it has some antioxidant compounds that protect the liver and, consequently, improve the entire digestive process. Also, served as an appetizer; the rocket can stimulate the appetite.

✓ It lowers the pressure. The consumption of arugula counteracts hypertension because the potassium it contains helps eliminate excess fluid, balancing blood pressure.

✓ It prevents tumors. This action is possible thanks to the good amount of antioxidants present in rocket such as beta-carotene, vitamin C, lutein, and zeaxanthin, but also flavonoids and isothiocyanates such as sulforaphane.

✓ It strengthens nails and bones. The calcium contained in arugula can help enhance the structure of nails and bones. Besides, as we have seen above, vitamin K has a protective effect on the bone system.

✓ Excellent in pregnancy: As we have seen, the arugula is rich in folates, which, by transforming into folic acid, have a preventive action against fetal malformations and is useful for the correct growth of the baby.

✓ It detoxifies the body: The high content of water and minerals and the presence of fibers give the rocket detoxifying properties, thus helping to expel toxins and harmful substances from the liver and kidneys.

✓ It is protective against ulcers: A 2009 study published in the World Journal of Gastroenterology found that a rocket extract was effective in mice in inhibiting acid secretion and stimulating mucus production that protects stomach walls, thus preventing the development of ulcers. The effect would be due to the antioxidants present in the arugula and prostaglandins with anti-inflammatory effects.

✓ It has a relaxing function. When taken as an infusion, the arugula has relaxing properties and is recommended to promote good sleep. It is part of some "evening herbal teas."

In general, it should be consumed fresh and after washing it well because it is in direct contact with the ground. If you want to keep it in the fridge, it is necessary to clean it and keep it in a paper bag after having dried it well.

Its consumption has no particular contraindications, except, of course, in allergy sufferers. It is always good not to consume too much of it because it could have irritating effects, especially on the gastrointestinal system. We did not recommend it for those who take anticoagulant drugs (for the high content of vitamin K), for those suffering from stones and kidney failure.

The rocket infusion can be used to promote relaxation. Just put six rocket leaves in a cup of boiling water and let it infuse for 10 minutes. To reduce the bitter taste of the rocket, we recommend adding a teaspoon of chamomile flowers.

※※※

Soy

- Sirtuin activator nutrients: daidzein and formononetin.

Miso, produced from fermented soybeans, is a traditional Japanese food. In addition to its fantastic health-promoting properties, the thing that makes it indispensable is its wonderful umami flavor, which gives an explosion of taste to your dishes.

Avoid those that contain sodium glutamate (MSG), an ingredient artificially created to reproduce its flavor.

Of Asian origin, soya was grown for food over 5000 years ago. The Chinese were already familiar with the properties of soybean, and it is listed in the first known medical book: *Pen Tsao Gong Mo*.

It is a plant belonging to the family of leguminous plants, has an erect stem that can reach up to 80/90 cm in height, and the fruits are flat pods, similar to our peas. A lot of derivatives of this legume are used nowadays: soy sauce, soy sprouts, soy milk, soy flour, from which as many varieties of food products are derived.

There are different types: yellow, black, red, and green. As far as red and green soya beans are concerned, it should be pointed out that they are azuki beans and mung beans, respectively, and both do not belong to the same botanical species as yellow soya (the Glycine max plant, which we typically identify as "soya"). Green soybeans are also used to produce soybean sprouts.

Soybeans harvested unripe, on the other hand, are called edamame.

Soya provides 446 calories per 100 grams. It is food particularly rich in proteins of high biological value, minerals and, like all legumes, offers the right amount of fiber, useful for the welfare of the intestine.

Soya beans contain proteins (about 36%) and fats (20%), the latter consisting mainly of unsaturated fatty acids, which play a fundamental role in our body: they play a preventive action against many alterations and diseases. This legume is also rich in minerals such as calcium, phosphorus, potassium, magnesium, and iron. There are also vitamins A and various B vitamins, including B1, B2, B3, B5, and B6. It also contains fiber that is well tolerated by our body, which helps fight constipation, regularizes blood sugar levels, and helps to normalize the level of cholesterol in the blood. This legume is also able to exert various beneficial effects on our body. It has been shown that soy lowers cholesterol, promotes bone mineralization by preventing osteoporosis, helps the digestive system in the case of lazy intestines, and helps in the prevention of cancer. Finally, thanks to Isoflavones, soy is an excellent remedy against menopause disorders because Isoflavones help to replenish part of the estrogen, no longer produced by the ovaries.

***

Strawberries

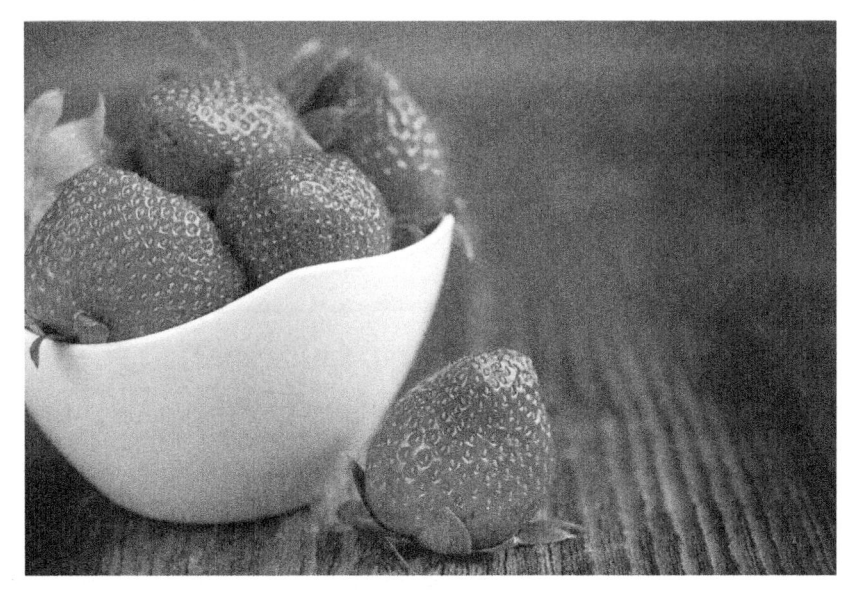

- Nutrient activators of sirtuin: fisetin.

Strawberries have a shallow sugar content (1 teaspoon per 100 g). Also, when added to foods that contain carbohydrates, they help reduce the body's insulin demand, transforming the food into a slow-release energy source. They should be an integral part of all slimming and healthy diets.

The antioxidants contained in strawberries (ellagic acid, vitamin C, and flavonoids) help to lose weight because they fight inflammations that prevent certain hormones from stimulating slimming. Also, these antioxidants in strawberries increase the production of a hormone called adiponectin, which boosts metabolism and reduces appetite and decrease starch absorption. Besides, they can control blood sugar levels and thus prevent diabetes and the formation of abdominal fat. In practice, consumed as part of a balanced diet, they allow the body to restore its natural ability to lose weight.

Some research has shown that strawberries have a high capacity to stimulate a natural mechanism that leads the brain to "self-clean, eliminating toxic substances that promote the reduction of brain functions, such as memory, and the appearance of dementia, including Alzheimer's, and Parkinson's disease. As time goes by, the accumulation of waste and toxins causes this mechanism to jam, and this causes damage to neurons. That is why, in a healthy and balanced diet, strawberries should not be missing!

The vitamin C content of strawberries (five fruits contain the same amount of vitamin C as an orange) promotes the production of collagen. This protein prevents wrinkles and strengthens capillaries by reducing water retention and cellulite. This anti-retention action is enhanced by potassium, a mineral-rich in strawberries.

If you water the strawberries in a tray, check that there are no dented or moldy fruits, because within a short time the mold can spread to the whole package. Choose the turgid strawberries with a bright, uniform red color and a petiole that is well attached to the fruit.

***

Turmeric

- Nutrient activators of sirtuin: turmeric.

It is believed that turmeric, also known as "Indian solid gold," is one of the factors contributing to the lower percentage of cancer patients in India, compared to Western countries. Studies have shown that a particular type of curcumin helps to improve cholesterol levels and control blood sugar levels, as well as reduce inflammation. Turmeric has also been shown to be an excellent natural painkiller in cases of knee arthrosis.

Turmeric is a spice rich in beneficial properties. For example, the consumption of turmeric improves the functioning of the stomach and intestines ,and also helps to combat cholesterol, since it facilitates the disposal of excess lipids. It has:

- Anti-inflammatory properties
- Antioxidant properties
- Choleretic properties
- Anti-tumor properties
- Healing properties
- Digestive properties
- Antidepressant properties
- Antibacterial properties
- Pain-relieving properties
- Detoxifying properties

Recognizing the benefits of turmeric to our health is now Western medicine, whose studies it has increasingly proved to be at the center of over the past few years.

Benefits:
- Prevents and reduces inflammation
- Relieves joint pain
- Benefits the brain and nervous system
- It's a natural painkiller
- Protects the liver
- Helps digestion
- Limits the action of free radicals
- Strengthens the immune system
- Prevents type 2 diabetes
- Helps the body to detoxify itself
- Prevents bacterial infections
- Promotes wound healing
- Contributes to the effectiveness of antidepressant drugs
- Increases memory
- Increases the self-healing capacity of the brain
- Helps prevent and fight tumors

***

Walnuts

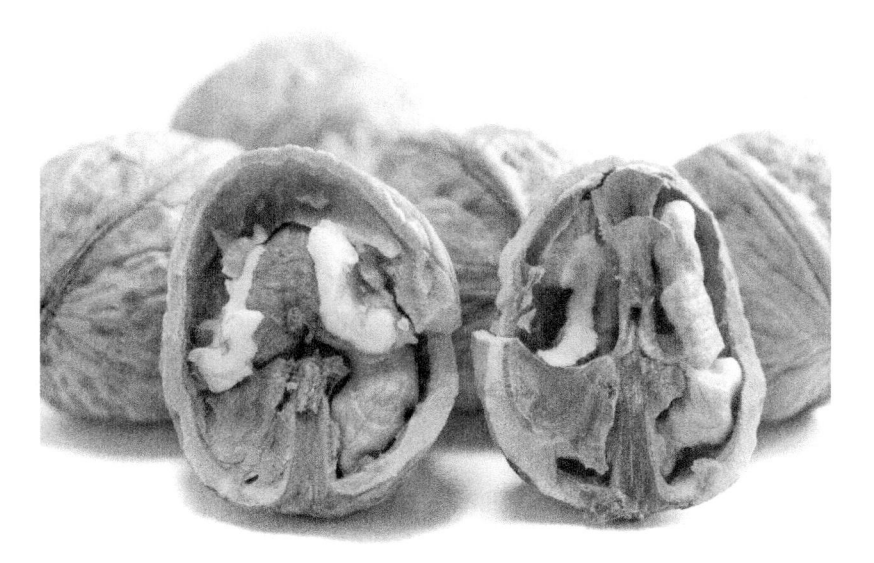

- Sirtuin activator nutrients: Gallic acid.

Walnuts undermine all traditional beliefs about food: they are rich in fat and high in calorie;, yet they have been widely proven to contribute to weight loss and improve certain metabolic disorders for the power of sirtuin activation.

Nuts are oval fruits covered with a green shell called a hull. When the walnut is fully ripe, the hull dries and blackens, causing the tree to fall off.

As there is a lot of moisture inside the hull, the walnuts need to be properly dried before being eaten. Inside the shell, we find the walnut kernels, which are the edible part. There are different varieties of walnuts. Very famous are the Californian walnuts, with the most massive shell. There are the Brazil walnuts, very rich in Selenium, a mineral that is a powerful antioxidant and therefore protects against the action of free radicals. The Pecan walnuts have the highest fat content and, therefore, calories, but rich in antioxidants that counteract aging. Al final, the Macadamia walnuts have a sweeter and more delicate taste and seem to have a powerful anti-aging effect.

The nuts contain essential nutrients, which have proven to be preventive against various diseases.

Walnuts are very caloric, and therefore, energetic fruits, providing about 650 calories per 100 gr of product. They are mostly made up of fats and proteins. The fats, however, are unsaturated and therefore have numerous health benefits, especially for the heart. Fibers are also present in the right quantity, helping in the regulation of intestinal functions; therefore, it is used in the case of constipation and balancing the levels of cholesterol and blood glucose.

Among the most abundant vitamins in nuts are the B vitamins; in particular, B1 and B6, but also vitamin E and folic acid. Among the minerals, we find mainly Calcium, Iron, Magnesium, but also Zinc, Phosphorus, and Potassium. Walnuts are also rich in monounsaturated and polyunsaturated fatty acids. Let's see in detail, which are the most abundant, and their related properties.

Monounsaturated and polyunsaturated fatty acids: the most present monounsaturated fatty acid is oleic acid, while among the polyunsaturated, we find fats from the Omega 3 and Omega 6 series. These fats are defined as essential because they are not produced by our bodies and must necessarily be taken through food. They are particularly beneficial for the cardiovascular system as they help to reduce levels of LDL cholesterol, the "bad" cholesterol that is deposited in the arteries, and triglycerides. The fatty acids Omega-3 and Omega-6 also have a valuable anti-inflammatory and anti-tumor action. For all these reasons they are called "good" fats.

Vitamin B1 or thiamine: it is a vitamin present in the right quantities in nuts and indispensable in energy metabolism. It regulates the functions of the nervous system but also of the heart and muscular system.

Vitamin B6: regulates the synthesis of serotonin, which prevents disorders such as depression and insomnia, regulates the functions of the immune system, and protects brain functions so that a deficiency of this vitamin can lead to neurological diseases such as Parkinson's disease. Folic acid or vitamin B9: is present in the right quantities in nuts. It is an essential compound for the production of hemoglobin, so it plays a crucial role both during growth and during pregnancy, avoiding the onset of fetal malformations.

Vitamin E: it is a precious antioxidant, which therefore protects against the damaging action of free radicals.

Calcium: it is fundamental for the health of bones and teeth but also the heart and muscular system.

Iron: it enters the constitution of hemoglobin, a protein that distributes oxygen to the tissues; its deficiency can lead to anemia, with consequent tiredness, paleness, and muscle cramps.

Magnesium: This mineral becomes part of various biological processes and restores the balance of the nervous system, lowers blood pressure, prevents cardiovascular diseases, and stimulates the functions of the muscular system.

Arginine: among the amino acids present in walnuts is arginine, which performs many fundamental functions. Arginine promotes the dilation of blood vessels, facilitates wound healing, contributes to the disposal of waste substances such as ammonia, and the formation of creatine, a substance that reduces recovery time after physical effort.

Walnuts are good from several points of view: The combination of the nutrients we have just seen gives nuts numerous health benefits; let's see them together.

✓ <u>Walnuts are suitable for the health of the heart</u>: Regularly eating nuts helps to prevent cardiovascular diseases such as heart attacks. As already mentioned, walnuts contain fats that can reduce cholesterolemia, which is beneficial for the health of the heart.

✓ <u>Anti-tumor properties</u>. This property of walnut is due to the presence of antioxidants and Omega 3 fatty acids. This action would occur mainly in breast and prostate cancer.

✓ <u>They are energetic and improve physical performance</u>: Thanks to their high energy power and the presence of proteins, magnesium, and arginine, walnuts are ideal for recovering energy in particularly demanding periods and for those who practice sports.

✓ <u>Walnuts counteract hypertension</u>. This property of nuts is due to polyunsaturated fatty acids, in particular alpha-linoleic acid, arginine, which increases the elasticity of blood vessels and magnesium, which regulates blood pressure values.

✓ <u>They prevent blood sugar spikes</u>. In walnuts are molecules that can stabilize blood sugar. They are, therefore, suitable food in case of glycemic changes.

✓ <u>Walnuts improve mood</u>. A regular consumption of nuts can improve mood, thanks to the presence of Omega-3, magnesium, and tryptophan. According to a recent study carried out by the University of New Mexico[3], young men in particular benefit from this effect. According to scholars, this effect is also attributable to vitamin E and melatonin.

To benefit from all the positive effects, just consume 6-7 nuts per day, corresponding to about 30 g of kernels. The ideal would be to eat them at breakfast, or in a snack. They can also be added to the salad to make it tasty and rich in properties. Thanks to its versatility, it can be added to any dish!

---

[3] https://news.unm.edu/news/the-key-to-a-better-mood-for-young-men-is-a-nut

CHAPTER 3 - THE GREEN JUICE

The green Sirtfood Diet juice is the *central* piece of the Sirtfood diet. Regardless of whether you are not aiming to follow the diet, the liquid is full of nutrients and would be a great choice towards a regular diet. It is a special centrifugate that can purify and satiate at the same time.

The first stage of the diet has this much juice as its focal food, which is green because of the ingredients it contains.

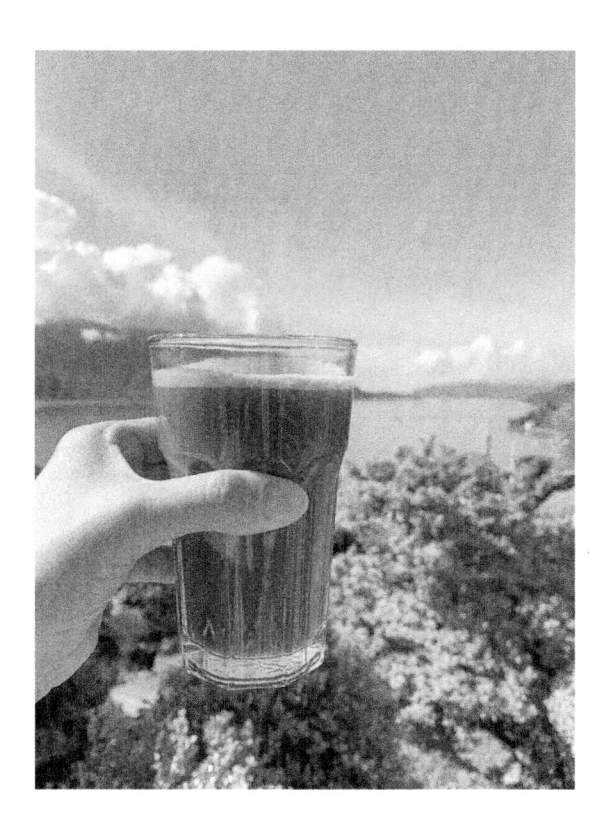

How to prepare green juice

Ingredients:

- 75g kale
- 30g rocket salad
- 5g parsley
- 2 celery sticks
- ½ green apple
- Juice of ½ lemon
- ½ teaspoon matcha green tea

It is prepared by centrifuging 75 grams of kale, 30 grams of rocket salad, and 5 grams of parsley.

Add 150 grams of green celery with leaves and half a green apple, both grated.

Finally, half squeezed lemon and half teaspoon of matcha tea will enrich the whole with antioxidants and vitamins.

This detox drink should preferably be prepared at the time of consumption, without storing it in the fridge, so as not to lose valuable benefits of the nutrients.

Options

If the taste is not pleasant, it is possible to make changes or add additional ingredients to make it tastier.
- ✓ Add a few mint leaves
- ✓ You can use a whole apple
- ✓ You can remove the parsley and add the strawberries
- ✓ You can drink water right after you drink it.
- ✓ Can be more pleasant cold, adding a little ice
- ✓ You can change the arugula with 1cm ginger

CHAPTER 4 – DIET PLAN

The First Phase

The Sirtfood diet, being a low-calorie diet, the first three days are particularly demanding: the daily calories are very few (1,000), and given almost only by Sirt food. The weekly scheme provides, in this first moment of attack, only one solid meal per day and three green Sirt juices.

In the following four days, on the other hand, the number of calories is increased to 1500 by adding a second substantial meal.

This first phase corresponds to a weight-loss of about 7 pounds.

Menu type:
- Breakfast: water + tea or espresso coffee + 1 cup of green juice;
- Lunch: green juice (3 cups total in a day);
- Snack: a square of dark chocolate;
- Dinner: buckwheat pasta + vegetables and chicken.
- After dinner: a square of dark chocolate.

The first three days are the hardest. The calories are just 1000. We are on a kind of lightfast, based mainly on juices, which encourages the body to eliminate waste from cells and consume fat. Hunger is kept under control, thanks to the abundance of Sirt food. Then, from the fourth to seventh day, calories rise to

1500, while centrifuges decrease to two. Al final, the solid meals increase to two.

Already from the first day, a piece of dark chocolate can be eaten. To earn the title of Sirt food, it must be chocolate with 85 percent cocoa. And even among the various types of chocolate with this percentage, not all of them are the same. Often this product is treated with an alkalizing agent (this is the so-called "Dutch process") to reduce its acidity and give it a darker color. Unfortunately, this process strongly reduces the flavonoid activators of sirtuin, compromising its health benefits. Therefore always, chocolate is not subject to the Dutch method.

Regarding the drinks that we suggest during the diet, let's not forget water, coffee, and tea.

We all know that green tea is right for your health, and water is, of course, fine, but what about coffee? More than half of people drink at least one cup of coffee a day, but always with a trace of guilt because they have led us to think that this is a vice and an unhealthy habit: nothing more false. Studies show that coffee is a real treasure trove of beneficial plant substances because coffee drinkers run less risk of diabetes, certain forms of cancer, and neurodegenerative diseases. Moreover, not only is coffee not a toxin, it also protects the liver and makes it healthier!

Before starting any diet, it is an excellent habit to take a frontal and profile photo. Another essential action is to mark all body measurements (chest, waist, and hips), to evaluate all progress.

The Second Phase

Phase 2 lasts about two weeks and is used to preserve and maintain the weight loss obtained in the first phase.

In this step, there is only one juice left, and the substantial "dishes" get to 3. There are more calorie restrictions but only indications on which foods to take Sirt.

> *1 green Sirt juices + 3 solid meal + 15-20g dark chocolate*

You have to stock up on curly kale, dark chocolate, red wine, citrus fruits, coffee, blueberries, capers, green tea, soy, and strawberries to maintain the results.

Those who need to lose more weight can repeat the diet every three months.

CHAPTER 5: THE FIRST PHASE: 7 POUNDS IN 7 DAYS

In this first phase, we will accompany you day by day, proposing recipes. You can also choose the recipes in the dedicated chapter.

7-Day Meal Plan

Day 1

The first day you will eat:

> *3 green juices Sirt + 1 solid meal + 15-20g of dark chocolate*

Drink the juices at three different times of the day (e.g., in the morning as soon as you wake up, mid-morning and mid-afternoon) and choose the standard or vegan dish.

And finally, 15-20g dark chocolate (85 percent cocoa).

Recipe 1 - *Prawns with buckwheat*

Serves 1

Ingredients:

- 150 g peeled prawns
- 1 teaspoon of tamari
- 2 teaspoons of extra virgin olive oil
- 75 g of buckwheat spaghetti
- 1 clove of garlic
- 1 chilli
- 1 teaspoon of ginger
- 20 g of red onion
- 40 g celery
- 75 g of chopped green beans,
- 50 g kale

Directions

Cook the shelled prawns for 2-3 minutes with one teaspoon of tamari and one teaspoon of extra virgin olive oil.

Boil the buckwheat spaghetti in water without salt, drain them and keep them aside.

Fry with another teaspoon of extra virgin olive oil, the clove of garlic, chilli pepper, and a teaspoon of finely chopped fresh ginger, sliced red onion, and celery, chopped green beans, and coarsely chopped kale.

Add 100 ml of water and bring to the boil leaving the vegetables to simmer while they are still crispy inside.

Add the prawns, spaghetti, and 5 g celery leaves, bring back to the boil, and serve.

Or Recipe 2- Turkey with cauliflower couscous

Serves 1

Ingredients:

- 150 g turkey
- 150 g of cauliflower tops
- 40 g of red onion
- 1 teaspoon of fresh ginger
- 1 Bird's-eye chilli
- 1 clove of garlic
- 3 teaspoons extra virgin olive oil
- 2 teaspoons of turmeric
- 30 g dried tomatoes
- 10 g parsley
- dried sage q.b.
- 1 tablespoon capers
- 1/4 fresh lemon juice

Directions

1. Blend the raw cauliflower tops and then cook them in a teaspoon of oil, garlic, red onion, chilli, ginger, and a teaspoon of turmeric, leave to flavor for a minute.

2. Add, over low heat, the chopped dried tomatoes and 5 g of parsley.

3. Season the turkey slice with one teaspoon of oil and the dried sage, and cook it in another teaspoon of oil.

4. Once ready, season with a tablespoon of capers, 1/4 of lemon juice, 5 g of parsley and a tablespoon of water, and add the cauliflower.

Day 2

> ***3 green juices Sirt + 1 solid meal + 15-20g of dark chocolate***

The formula is identical to that of the first day, and the only thing that changes is the solid meal. You'll have dark chocolate today too, and the same goes for tomorrow. This food is so excellent that we don't need an excuse to eat it.

On day 2, capers are also on the menu. They are not fruits, but buds that grow in Mediterranean countries and are picked by hand. They are fantastic Sirt foods because they are very rich in the nutrients kaempferol and quercitin. For taste, they are tiny concentrates of flavor. If you've never used them, don't be intimidated. You will see, they will drive you crazy if combined with the right ingredients, and they will give an unmistakable and inimitable aroma to your dishes.

Recipe 3 - Chicken with red onion and kale

Serves 1

Ingredients:

- 120 g chicken breast
- 130 g of tomatoes
- 1 Bird's-eye chilli
- 1 tablespoon capers
- 5 g parsley
- lemon juice
- 2 teaspoons of extra virgin olive oil
- 2 teaspoons of turmeric
- 50 g kale
- 20 g of red onion
- 1 teaspoon of fresh ginger
- 50 g of buckwheat

Directions

1. Marinate the chicken breast for 10 minutes with 1/4 lemon juice, 1 teaspoon of oil, and one teaspoon of turmeric powder.

2. Cut 130 g of tomatoes into chunks, remove the inner part, season with chilli pepper, one tablespoon capers, 1 teaspoon turmeric and one teaspoon oil, juice of 1/4 lemon, and 5 g chopped parsley.

3. cook the drained chicken breast over high heat for one minute on each side and then put it in the oven for about 10 minutes at 220°. Leave it to rest covered with aluminum foil.

4. steam the chopped cabbage for 5 minutes; in a pan fry the red onion, a teaspoon of freshly grated ginger and a teaspoon of oil; add the boiled cabbage and leave to flavor together for one minute over the heat.

5. Boil the buckwheat with turmeric, drain and serve with chicken, tomatoes, and chopped cabbage.

Or Recipe 4 – *Vegetable and buckwheat soup*

Serves 2

Ingredients:

- 200 g potatoes
- 200 g kohlrabi
- 100 g carrots
- 1 celery coast
- 1 red onion
- 500 ml of vegetable broth
- 1 tablespoon of extra virgin olive oil
- 2 cloves of garlic
- Halls
- 4 sage leaves
- 80 g of buckwheat
- 30 g of cheese
- 50 g of peeled red lentils

Directions

Wash the potatoes and kohlrabi, peel them, and cut them into cubes about an inch to the side.

Wash the carrots, peel them and slice them about 4 millimeters thick.

Wash the celery, remove the filaments and leaves, cut the rib into small cubes.

Peel the onion, cut it into quarters, then slice it to a thickness of 3-4 millimeters.

Heat the broth.

Put the oil and peeled garlic in a soup pot. Bring it to the heat and brown the garlic over a high flame.

Remove it, add all the vegetables, and cook stirring for a couple of minutes.

Add the stock, keeping some aside for the end of cooking, a pinch of salt, the sage leaves well washed, put the lid on, and wait for it to boil.

Cook for 15 minutes after it starts boiling again over medium heat, covered.

After the indicated time, taste, and add salt regularly. The cooking stock must be a little tasty.

Rinse the buckwheat and lentils under freshwater, then add them to the pot.

Cook for 20 minutes over medium heat. Cook with the lid on if you want a more liquid soup, and without, if you want it thicker.

Al final, taste, and add salt regularly.

Turn off the heat, add the Parmesan cheese, stir well and let it rest, and covered for a couple of minutes. If the soup is too thick, add some of the stock set aside.

Serve with a drizzle of raw oil.

Day 3

> *3 green juices Sirt + 1 solid meal + 15-20g of dark chocolate*

You are now on day three, and even though the format is identical to days 1 and 2, it's time to add a little flavor to the whole thing. For thousands of years, chilli pepper has been a fundamental element of gastronomic experiences around the world. As far as the health effects are concerned, we have already seen that its hotness is fantastic for activating the sirtuins and stimulating the metabolism. The applications of chilli peppers in the kitchen are endless, so they are easy ways to consume Sirt food regularly. While we know that not everyone likes spicy or spicy food, we hope at least to be able to convince you to use small amounts of it. It has been shown that those who eat spicy food at least three times a week have a 14 percent lower mortality rate than those who eat tasty food less than once a week. Our favorite hot pepper is Bird's Eye (sometimes called Thai chilli) because it is the best for sirtuins.

This is the last day you will consume three green juices a day. Tomorrow you will switch to two.

Recipe 5 - Pasta with smoked salmon with chilli and rocket

Ingredients for 4 servings

- 2 tablespoons of extra virgin olive oil
- 1 red onion, finely chopped
- 2 cloves of garlic, finely chopped
- 2 Bird's Eye chilli peppers, finely chopped
- 150g cherry tomatoes, cut in half
- 100ml white wine
- 250-300g buckwheat pasta
- 250g smoked salmon
- 2 tablespoons of capers
- 1/2 lemon juice
- 60g rocket salad
- 10g parsley, minced

Directions

Heat 1 teaspoon of oil in a pan over medium heat. Add the onion, garlic, and chilli, and fry until the ingredients are withered, but not dark.

Add the tomatoes and leave to cook for a minute or two. Pour in the white wine and let it simmer until it reduces by half.

Cook the pasta in boiling water with one teaspoon of oil for 8-10 minutes, depending on whether you prefer it more or less al dente, and drain.

Cut the salmon into strips and transfer it to the tomato pot with capers, lemon juice, rocket, and parsley.

Add the pasta, stir well, and serve immediately. Sprinkle with any remaining oil.

Or Recipe 6 – Buckwheat and tofu salad

The tofu and buckwheat salad is a delicious and tasty vegan summer recipe. This cold dish is perfect to be eaten at the beach, or in the office during the working lunch break.

Served strictly cold, the tofu, and buckwheat salad is a healthy, light, and nutritionally well-balanced dish. Thanks to the mineral salts, the proteins, and fibers of buckwheat and the vegetable proteins of tofu, this dish can also be easily served as a single dish. It is suitable to be eaten on hot days, the tofu and buckwheat salad will also be appreciated for its different consistencies.

Ingredients

- 300 gr of buckwheat
- 400 gr of cherry tomatoes
- 125 gr of natural tofu
- 3 tufts of basil
- 150 gr of sunflower seeds
- Evo oil q.b.
- Salt q.b.

Directions

Rinse the buckwheat under running water, put it in a pot full of cold water and cook for about twenty minutes; in the meantime, carefully wash the basil and tomatoes; cut the tomatoes into segments and put them in a large bowl.

When cooked, drain the buckwheat and cool it under running water, then add it to the tomatoes; add the crumbled or chopped tofu, break up the basil and add the sunflower seeds, the season is fine with oil and salt, and mix everything.

You can also serve it immediately or after it has cooled well in the refrigerator.

How to store tofu and buckwheat salad:

You can store this salad in the refrigerator for a couple of days, but only if stored in airtight containers.

Day 4

> *2 green Sirt juices + 2 solid meals + 15-20g of dark chocolate*

The fourth day of the Sirt diet has arrived, and you are halfway through your journey to a leaner, healthier body. The significant change from the previous three days is that you will only drink two juices instead of three, and you will have two solid meals instead of one. For today and the other days that remain, that means two green juices and two delicious, solid meals rich in Sirt food. The inclusion of Medjoul dates in a list of foods that promote slimming and good health may seem surprising to you. Especially when you think that they contain as much as 66 percent sugar.

Sugar has no stimulant properties towards sirtuins. On the contrary, it has well-known links with obesity, heart disease, and diabetes; in short, just the opposite of what we are aiming for. But refined and industrially processed sugar is very different from sugar present in a food that also contains polyphenols that activate sirtuins: Medjoul dates. Unlike regular sugar, these dates, consumed in moderation, do not increase blood glucose levels.

Recipe 7 - Chocolate Tartufini Sirt

Ingredients for 15-20 truffles

- 120g walnuts
- 30g dark chocolate (85 per cent cocoa), broken into pieces, or crushed cocoa beans
- 250g Medjoul dates, deprived of the seed
- 1 tablespoon of cocoa powder
- 1 tablespoon turmeric powder
- 1 tablespoon of extra virgin olive oil
- seeds of 1 vanilla pod or 1 teaspoon of vanilla extract
- 1-2 tablespoons of water

Directions:

Put the nuts and chocolate in a food processor and blend until a fine powder is obtained. Add all the other ingredients minus the water and blend until the mixture cures into a ball. You may have to add water, but it depends on the consistency of the mix, which should not be too sticky.

Using your hands, form balls the size of walnuts and put them in the fridge in a sealed container at least 1 hour before eating them. You can dip them in cocoa or dried coconut flakes to give them a slightly different taste. They will keep in the fridge for a week at most.

Today we will also integrate red chicory into the meals. Like the onion, the red quality is better, but endive, a close relative of the onion, is also a Sirt food. If you are looking for ideas on how to use these salads, combine them with other varieties and dress them with olive oil: they will give a spicy taste to milder leaves.

Or Recipe 8 - Waldorf Salad

Ingredients:

- 1 portion 100g celery, coarsely chopped
- 50g apple, coarsely chopped
- 50g walnuts, coarsely chopped
- 10g red onion, coarsely chopped
- 5g chopped parsley
- 1 tablespoon capers
- 5g of lovage or celery leaves, coarsely chopped
- 1 tablespoon of extra virgin olive oil
- 1 tablespoon balsamic vinegar
- 1/4 lemon juice
- the tip of a teaspoon of Dijon mustard
- 50g arugula
- 35g red chicory leaves

Directions

Mix celery, apple, walnuts, onion, parsley, capers, and lovage or celery leaves. In a bowl, mix the oil, vinegar, lemon juice, and mustard and work everything with whips to obtain the seasoning.

Place the celery mixture on the rocket and red chicory and pour over the sauce.

Day 5

> *2 green Sirt juices + 2 solid meals + 15-20g of dark chocolate*

You have reached day five, and it is time to add some fruit. Due to its high sugar content, the fruit has poorly been advertised, but this does not apply to berries. Strawberries have a shallow sugar content: one teaspoon per 100 grams. They also have an excellent effect on the way the body processes simple sugars. Scientists have found that if we add strawberries to simple sugars, this causes a reduction in insulin demand, and thus turns the food into a machine that releases energy over a long period. Strawberries are, therefore, a perfect element in diets that aim to lose weight and want to get you back into shape. They are also delicious and extremely versatile, as you will discover in the Sirt version of the fresh and light Middle Eastern tabbouleh.

Miso, made from fermented soya, is a traditional Japanese dish. Miso has a strong umami taste, a real explosion for the taste buds. In our modern society, we know better the monosodium glutamate, artificially created to reproduce the same taste. It is far preferable to derive that magical umami taste from a traditional, natural food full of beneficial substances. It is found in the form of pasta in all good supermarkets and natural food stores and should be present in every kitchen to give a touch of taste to many different dishes. As the umami flavors reinforce each other, miso is perfectly combined with other tasty/human foods, especially when it comes to cooked protein, as you will discover today in the savory, fast and easy dishes we are about to offer you.

Recipe 9 - Buckwheat pancakes with strawberries and chocolate

Ingredients for 6-8 pancakes

For pancakes
- 350ml of milk
- 150g buckwheat flour
- 1 big egg
- 1 tablespoon of extra virgin olive oil
- For the chocolate sauce:
- 100g dark chocolate (85 percent cocoa).
- 85ml of milk
- 1 tablespoon double cream
- 1 tablespoon of extra virgin olive oil

For garnish:
- 400g strawberries, peeled and chopped.
- 100g of chopped walnuts

Directions:

To prepare the pancakes, pour all the ingredients minus the oil into a blender and blend until the dough is smooth, not too dense or too liquid. (You can store the excess in an airtight container in the refrigerator for up to 5 days. Make sure you mix it well before using it). To prepare the sauce, melt the chocolate in a bowl on a pot of boiling water. When it is melted, add the milk, stirring well, then the cream and olive oil. You can keep it warm by leaving it on the pot over a very low flame until the pancakes are ready.

Pour mixture in the pan, and move it by tilting it so that it is spread all over the surface. If necessary, add a little more of the mixture. It will take about a minute to cook on each side. When the edges become brownish, use a spatula to lift the pancake along the outer perimeter and turn it. Try to do this with a single movement to avoid breaking it. Cook it on the other side for a minute and transfer it to a tray.

Place some strawberries in the middle and roll up the pancake. Continue until you've made all the pancakes you want.

Or Recipe 10 - Pumpkin soup

Ingredients:

- 1500g pumpkin
- 1 tablespoon of miso
- 1 Lemon
- 1 Orange
- Red onion
- Extra virgin olive oil
- Salt q.b.

Directions

Choose a pumpkin with firm flesh.

With half a pumpkin (about 1.5 kg) you will get 4 portions.

Cut it into large pieces and put it directly into the oven without any seasoning. Cook until soft (about 40 minutes at 180° in ventilated mode): in this way, the outer part will roast slightly and will leave a great taste. Once cooked, let it cool and then peel it. In the meantime, lower the oven to about 50 degrees.

Remove the peel (only the colored part, not the white skin) with half a lemon and about ¼ of orange - if you had a cedar, it would be even better - and put it in the oven to dry (about 10 minutes). Once dry, chop it.

In a pan, brown the onion in vegetable oil; add the pumpkin pulp, stretch it with two glasses of water, and blend it all. Add the citrus peel and a generous spoonful of miso. Let it simmer until the miso is melted and the ingredients mixed. Add salt and serve warm.

Day 6

> ***2 green Sirt juices + 2 solid meals + 15-20g of dark chocolate***

There is no Sirt food better than olive oil and red wine. Virgin olive oil is obtained from the fruit only by mechanical means, in conditions that do not deteriorate it, so that you can be sure of its quality and polyphenol content. The "extra virgin" oil is that of the first pressing ("virgin" is the fruit of the second one) and therefore has more taste and better quality: this is what we strongly suggest you use.

No Sirt menu would be complete without red wine, one of the cornerstones of the diet. It contains sirtuins resveratrol and piceatannol activators, which probably explain the longevity and slimness associated with the traditional French way of life, and which are at the origin of the enthusiasm triggered by Sirt foods. Of course, wine contains alcohol, so it should be consumed in moderation. But luckily, resveratrol can withstand heat well so that it can be used in the kitchen. Pinot Noir is our favorite grape variety because it contains much more resveratrol than the others.

Recipe 11 - Chicken breast with walnut and parmesan pesto and red onion

Serves 1

Ingredients:

- 15g parsley
- 15g pecans
- 4 teaspoons (15g) Parmesan cheese, minced
- 1 tablespoon of virgin olive oil
- 1/2 lemon juice
- 3 tablespoons (50ml) of water
- 150g chicken breast without the skin
- 20g red onions, finely chopped
- 1 teaspoon of red wine vinegar
- 35g rocket
- 100g split cherry tomatoes
- 1 teaspoon of balsamic vinegar

Directions:

Put the parsley, pecans, parmesan, parmesan, olive oil, most of the lemon juice, and some water in a food processor or blender and stir until smooth. Include more water slowly until the desired consistency is obtained. Marinate the chicken breast in 1 tablespoon of pesto and the rest of the lemon juice in the cooler for 30 minutes; longer if possible. Preheat the stove to 392°F

(200°C). Heat an oven-proof pan with medium to high heat. Fry the marinated chicken on both sides, then move it to the oven and cook for 8 minutes, or until fully cooked. Marinate the onions in red wine vinegar for 5-10 minutes. When the chicken is cooked, remove it from the plate, put another spoonful of pesto on it and let the pesto melt with the heat of the chicken. Let it rest for 5 minutes before serving. Add the rocket, tomatoes, and onion; and sprinkle with balsamic vinegar.

Or Recipe 12 - Meat and chilli

Serves: 4

Ingredients:
- 1 red onion, finely chopped
- 3 cloves of garlic, finely chopped
- 2 Thai chilli peppers, finely chopped
- 1 tablespoon of additional virgin olive oil
- 1 tablespoon of ground cumin
- 1 tablespoon of ground turmeric
- 450g ground lean hamburger (5 percent fat)
- 150ml of red wine
- 1 chilli pepper, with core, semi-evacuated and cut into small pieces
- 400g jars of cut tomatoes

- 1 tablespoon of tomato puree
- 1 tablespoon of cocoa powder
- 150g canned beans
- 300ml meat broth
- 2 tablespoons (5g) of new, cut coriander
- 2 tablespoons (5g) fresh parsley, chopped
- 1 cup (160g) of buckwheat

Directions

In a huge pot, fry the onion, garlic, and bean stew in oil over medium heat for 2 or 3 minutes, then include the flavors and cook for another moment or two. Include the ground hamburger and cook for 2 or 3 minutes over medium-high heat until the meat is nicely caramelized everywhere. Include the red wine and let it rise to decrease significantly. Include the red pepper, tomatoes, tomato puree, cocoa, beans, and broth and leave to stew for 60 minutes. You can include a little water from time to time to get a thick, sticky consistency. Not long before serving, stir in the cut herbs. In the meantime, cook the buckwheat as indicated in the bundle guidelines and serve near the stew.

Day 7

> ***2 green Sirt juices + 2 solid meals + 15-20g of dark chocolate***

With this day, you conclude the first phase. In this week, you should have weigh-lost about 7 pounds already. Most of the weight you've lost is through all the liquid you've accumulated, but that's an excellent start.

Today you can delight yourself with a particular recipe, the Sirt-pizza!

Recipe 13 - *Pizza Sirt*

(for two pizzas of 30cm)

For the pizza base:
- 1 pack of 7g dry yeast
- 1 teaspoon of brown sugar
- 300ml of lukewarm water
- 200g buckwheat flour
- 200g strong white flour or type 00
- 1 tablespoon of extra virgin olive oil, and a little more for oiling

For the tomato sauce:

- 1/2 red onion, finely chopped
- 1 clove of garlic, finely chopped
- 1 teaspoon of extra virgin olive oil
- 1 teaspoon of dried oregano
- 2 tablespoons of white wine
- 1 jar of 400g of tomato puree
- 1 pinch of brown sugar
- 5g basil leaves

Directions

Ideas for seals:

- Rocket, red onion, and grilled eggplant.

Heat a plate until it starts smoking, then reduce the temperature by adjusting the stove to a medium flame. Slice eggplant in 3-5mm slices, brush them with a little extra virgin olive oil, and cook until you have black marks on both sides of the eggplant, and the pieces are nice and soft. Alternatively, you can bake it in the oven on a baking tray covered with baking paper, at 200°C, for 15 minutes, or until it is soft and well browned).

- Chilli flakes, cherry tomatoes, goat cheese and arugula
- Chicken already cooked, rocket, red onion, and olives
- Cooked chorizo, red onion, and steamed kale

For the dough:

Dissolve the yeast and sugar in water: This will help activate the yeast. Sift the flour into a bowl. (If you have a food processor, put the kneading hook and pour the flour dough into the bowl provided).

Pour the yeast and oil mixture into the flour and knead. You may need to add a little water if the mix is too dry. Work until the mixture is homogeneous and elastic. Transfer it to an oiled bowl, cover with a clean damp cloth and leave to rise in a warm place for 45-60 minutes, until it has doubled in volume.

In the meantime, prepare the tomato sauce. Fry the onion and garlic in olive oil, then add the oregano. Add the wine and simmer until it reduces by half.

Add the tomato puree and sugar, bring to the boil and cook for 30 minutes until the sauce is thick. Break the basil leaves into pieces and add them to the sauce.

Heat the oven to 230°C (446°F).

Cut the dough in half and roll out both pieces of dough on a pizza stone or non-stick baking sheet until the desired thickness is reached.

Spread a thin layer of tomato sauce on the surface (you only need half of the sauce for this amount of dough, but you can freeze what remains), avoiding a fine strip along the edge. Add the rest of the ingredients (if you are using rocket and chilli flakes, add them after cooking). Let it rest about 15-20 minutes before baking, so the dough will rise a little more, becoming lighter.

Bake in the oven for 10-12 minutes or until the cheese is golden brown.

If you use them, add the arugula and chilli flakes at the end of cooking.

Or Recipe 14 - Buckwheat pasta salad

Ingredients:

- 50g of buckwheat pasta
- 1 large handful of arugula
- 1 handful of basil leaves
- 8 cherry tomatoes, cut in half
- 1/2 diced avocados
- 10 olives
- 1 tablespoon of extra virgin olive oil
- 20g pine nuts

Directions

Gently mix all the ingredients except the pine nuts and place them on a plate, then spread the pine nuts on top.

CHAPTER 6: THE SECOND PHASE: MAINTENANCE

The second phase of the diet lasts two weeks and consolidates the weight loss achieved in the first.

Remember:

> *1 green Sirt juices + 3 solid meal + 15-20g dark chocolate*

RECIPES

For the second phase, you can choose the recipe you wish.

Recipe 15 - Buckwheat and broccoli with chickpeas

Serves 2

Ingredients:
- 100 g of buckwheat
- 150 g of cooked chickpeas
- 1 Roman cabbage
- 1 red onion
- 3 tablespoons of low-fat yogurt
- 1 cm of ginger root
- 2 tablespoons of extra virgin olive oil

- salt and pepper to taste
- 1 teaspoon of turmeric powder

Directions

Boil the cabbage florets in salted water for 10 minutes; in the meantime, toast the buckwheat (left to soak for a couple of hours) in a non-stick pan for about 5 minutes, then boil it in the cabbage cooking water (after draining them) for 15-20 minutes.

In a separate pan, fry the onion and ginger root in 2 tablespoons of oil, add the cabbage florets, the cooked chickpeas, and finally the buckwheat, letting it cook for a few minutes. Turn it off, and if you like, accompany the dish with a yogurt sauce prepared by mixing the turmeric with the yogurt, adding a pinch of salt and pepper.

Recipe 16 - Buckwheat meatballs.

Serves 2/4

Ingredients:

- 100 grams of buckwheat;
- 1 whole egg;
- a clove of garlic;
- a bunch of parsley;
- nutmeg;
- breadcrumbs;
- salt and pepper.

Directions:

Wash the buckwheat and transfer it to a pot. Let it toast for a few seconds, after which add about 250/300 ml of cold water, add a pinch of salt, and cook for about 20-25 minutes. Chop a clove of garlic and put it in a pan with a drizzle of oil, add the buckwheat well drained from the remaining cooking water and let it flavor together for a few minutes. Transfer everything into a bowl and let it cool.

When the wheat is warm, add the slightly beaten egg, nutmeg, finely chopped parsley, a pinch of pepper, and mix well.

Cooking:

Now form some balls with the help of a spoon and roll them in breadcrumbs. Compact the meatballs by squeezing them between the palms of your hands and, at the same time, flatten them slightly at the poles. Grease a pan with oil and cook the meatballs on both sides until they are golden brown. Serve them hot buckwheat meatballs accompanied by vegetables to taste.

Recipe 17 - Cabbage and buckwheat fritters

Broccoli and buckwheat fritters are a tasty preparation for singles that are prepared by cooking the chopped shallot with broccoli in a pressure cooker; then the buckwheat will be added and at the end of cooking the mixture will be added to the flour. The meatballs will be obtained crushed and will be fried and served immediately on the table.

Ingredients:

- 20 g grated cheese
- 50 g cabbage tops
- 1 egg
- 1 tablespoon Flour 00
- 1/2 shallot
- Extra virgin olive oil
- Salt

Directions:

Clean the cabbage and choose the florets. Finely chop the shallot and put it in the pressure cooker with 1 tablespoon of oil and the cabbage florets.

Brown gently, add the buckwheat and twice as much saltwater or vegetable broth. Close the pan and cook for 15 minutes from the start of the hiss.

Open the pot and let the mixture cool down. Add the egg and add enough flour to obtain a homogeneous mixture with a moderately firm consistency.

If necessary, add salt to taste. With floured hands, form round meatballs and then crush them slightly to flatten them.

Place them in a baking tray and brush them with a drizzle of oil. Bake them in the oven for 15 minutes at about 200 °C (392 °F)

Recipe 18 - Buckwheat salad with artichokes

Serves: 4

Ingredients:
- 300 g buckwheat
- 200 g cherry tomatoes
- 5 artichokes
- 1 clove of garlic
- 1/2 cup large green olives
- fresh marjoram
- 5 tablespoons extra virgin olive oil
- salt
- 1 lemon

Directions:

In a non-stick pan, toast the buckwheat grains, always stirring for 3 or 4 minutes, then boil it in plenty of salted water for 10 minutes. It must remain very al dente. Drain and set aside.

Clean the artichokes: remove the outer leaves, trim them and remove the beard, cut them into segments, and throw them away as they are cleaned in water acidulated with lemon juice, so that they do not blacken.

In the meantime, brown the clove of garlic dressed lightly crushed in two tablespoons of oil.

When the artichokes are all hulled and cut, drain them and put them in the pan. Brown them without burning, then lower the heat and cook until they have softened a bit; they must remain al dente. Remove the garlic clove and sprinkle with a little fresh marjoram.

Put the buckwheat in the pan with the artichokes, stir well, and cook for a couple of minutes to make it taste good. Turn off and set aside.

Wash and cut the cherry tomatoes in half, leaving them a little in a colander to drain the vegetation water.

Cut the olives in half and remove the stone.

 Incorporate the cherry tomatoes and olives with buckwheat, add more marjoram leaves, stir and let them flavor well covered, over low heat.

Recipe 19 - Pasta with rocket salad and linseed

Serves: 4

Ingredients:

- 400 gr of wholemeal pasta
- 1 bunch of washed and dried Rocket
- 1 tablespoon of peeled almonds
- 1 tablespoon Linseed
- 1/2 clove of Garlic
- 4 spoons of extra virgin olive oil
- 3 tablespoons of water (if necessary)
- A few drops of lemon juice
- Salt
- Pepper

Directions:

First, wash the arugula and put it to dry on a kitchen cloth, then bring a pot of water to boil and throw the dough;

In a mixer, add 1 tablespoon of linseed, 1 tablespoon of almonds, half a clove of garlic (without the sprout) and 4 tablespoons of oil;

Cut everything for a few minutes, if necessary add a little water to make the pesto more fluid;

At this point add the rocket, a few drops of lemon juice, a pinch of salt and turn the mixer again for a few seconds, then add salt and pepper, and your pesto is ready;

Before draining the pasta, set aside some cooking water so that it can be used later, in case the pesto is too thick;

Once drained, put the pasta on the pot, season it with the pesto, and, if necessary, add a little cooking water previously-stored; continuing to stir for about a minute, and now your dish is ready to taste!

Recipe 20 - Rocket and strawberry salad

Serves: 1

Ingredients

- 1 tuft of rocket
- 8 champignon mushrooms
- 12 strawberries
- 1 tablespoon of extra virgin olive oil
- half a teaspoon of mustard
- salt
- pepper
- lemon juice

Directions

Wash and dry the rocket, then break the leaves into a bowl. Clean and slice the mushrooms and 8 ripe and firm strawberries. Also, put these ingredients in the bowl with the rocket. Mash 4 more strawberries well, add one tablespoon of extra virgin olive oil, half a teaspoon of mustard, salt, pepper, lemon juice, and emulsify with care. Pour the sauce over the salad, stir and serve.

Recipe 21 – Sirt Meat & chilli

for 4 servings

Ingredients

- 1 red onion, finely chopped
- 3 cloves of garlic, finely chopped
- 2 Bird's Eye chilli peppers, finely chopped
- 1 tablespoon of extra virgin olive oil
- 1 tablespoon of cumin powder
- 1 tablespoon turmeric powder
- 400g of ground lean beef (5% fat)
- 150ml of red wine
- 1 red pepper deprived of the stalks and seeds and cut into pieces
- 2 jars of 400g of peeled tomatoes
- 1 tablespoon of tomato paste
- 1 tablespoon of cocoa powder
- 150g canned beans
- 300ml beef broth
- 5g of chopped coriander

- 5g chopped parsley
- 160g buckwheat

Directions

In a saucepan, fry onion, garlic, and chilli pepper in oil, over medium heat for 2-3 minutes. Add the spices and cook for another minute or two. Add the minced meat and cook for another 2 or 3 minutes over medium-high heat until well browned. Pour in the red wine and simmer until it reduces by half.

Add the pepper, peeled tomatoes, tomato paste, cocoa, beans, and broth, and simmer for 1 hour. You may have to add a little water from time to time to get a thick sweet sauce. Add the chopped herbs just before serving. Cook the buckwheat according to the instructions on the package and serve with the chilli.

Recipe 22 - Sirt Eggs

1 portion

Ingredients

- 1 teaspoon of extra virgin olive oil
- 20g red onion, finely chopped
- 1/2 Bird's Eye chilli, finely chopped
- 3 average eggs 50ml milk

- 1 teaspoon of turmeric powder
- 5g parsley, finely chopped

Heat the oil in a frying pan and fry the onion and chilli pepper until soft, but do not let them darken.

Beat the eggs, milk, turmeric, and parsley. Pour into the hot pan and cook over medium-low heat, continuing to move the eggs to scramble, and prevent them from sticking and burning.

Serve when you have obtained the desired consistency.

Recipe 23 – Sirt Yogurt

1 portion

Ingredients

- 125g mixed berries
- 150g Greek yogurt
- 25g of chopped walnuts
- 10g of dark chocolate (85 percent cocoa) grated

Put your favorite berries in a bowl and pour yogurt on top. Sprinkle them with nuts and chocolate.

For a vegan alternative, you can replace Greek yogurt with soy or coconut milk.

Recipe 24 – Sirt pita bread

Whole grain pitas are an excellent way to fill up your Sirt food in a practical, fast, and easily transportable way. You can vary the quantities and have fun with the combinations, but the important thing is that you end up with a nice pita filled with excellent ingredients.

Ingredients

- 1 whole pita bread

Version with meat:

- 80g turkey sliced, minced
- 20g of diced Cheddar (or other cheese)
- 35g diced cucumbers
- 30g of chopped red onion
- 25g of chopped rocket
- 10-15g of coarsely chopped walnuts

For the sauce:

- 1 tablespoon of extra virgin olive oil
- 1 tablespoon balsamic vinegar
- a splash of lemon juice

Vegan version:

- 2-3 tablespoons of hummus
- 35g diced cucumbers
- 30g of chopped red onion
- 25g of chopped rocket
- 10-15g of coarsely chopped walnuts

Vegan sauce:

- 1 tablespoon of extra virgin olive oil
- a splash of lemon juice

Recipe 25 – Sirt Omelette

1 portion

Ingredients:

- 50g striped bacon (smoked or natural, according to taste)
- 3 medium eggs
- 35g red radicchio, finely sliced
- 5g parsley, finely chopped
- 1 teaspoon of extra virgin olive oil

Directions

Warm-up a non-stick frying pan. Cut the bacon into strips and fry it over a high flame until crispy—no need to add oil, just the bacon fat. Remove from the heat and place it on a sheet of kitchen paper to dry the excess fat. Clean the pan.

Beat the eggs and add the radicchio and parsley. Cut up the fried bacon and add it to the eggs. Heat the oil in the non-stick pan, which should be hot, but not steaming. Add the egg mixture and, using a spatula, move them to obtain smooth cooking. Reduce the flame and let the omelet harden. Lift it along the edges with the wooden spatula and fold it in half, or roll it up and serve.

Recipe 26 – Red bean sauce with baked potato

1 portion

Ingredients:

- 40g red onion, finely chopped
- 1 teaspoon of fresh ginger, finely chopped
- 1 clove of garlic, finely chopped
- 1 Bird's Eye chilli pepper, finely chopped
- 1 teaspoon of extra virgin olive oil
- 1 teaspoon of turmeric powder
- 1 teaspoon of cumin powder
- 1 pinch of powdered cloves
- 1 pinch of cinnamon powder
- 1 medium potato 190g peeled
- 1 teaspoon of brown sugar
- 50g red pepper, stripped of stalks and seeds and coarsely chopped
- 150ml vegetable stock
- 1 tablespoon of cocoa powder
- 1 teaspoon of sesame seeds
- 2 teaspoons of peanut butter (the velvety one is better, but the crunchy one is fine too)
- 150g canned red beans
- 5g chopped parsley

Directions

Heat the oven to 200 °C (392 °F).

Fry the onion, ginger, garlic, and chilli pepper in oil in a medium pan over medium heat for about 10 minutes, or until the ingredients have withered. Add the spices and cook for another 1-2 minutes.

Place the potato on a baking tray, put it in the hot oven and cook for 45-60 minutes until it is soft on the inside (or even longer if you like it crunchy on the outside).

Add the peeled tomatoes, sugar, peppers, stock, cocoa powder, sesame seeds, peanut butter, and beans; and simmer for 45-60 minutes.

Finally, sprinkle with parsley.

Recipe 27 – Tuna turkey

For Vegetable Bouillon:

- 2 potatoes
- 1 red onion
- 2 carrots
- 1 celery stalk
- Salt
- Pepper
- 1 tablespoon Extra virgin olive oil

For the meat:

- 800g Turkey breast
- 1 carrot
- 1 celery
- ½ red onion
- 1 bay leaf
- Juniper berries
- Salt
- Pepper
- 1 rosemary sprig

For the tuna sauce:

- 200g canned tuna
- 2 eggs
- 5 anchovy fillets
- 1 tablespoon capers

Directions

The tuna turkey, also called tonnè, is a second meat dish very simple to prepare. We use turkey meat, less fatty, but still very tasty. The homemade tuna sauce softens the turkey giving it an unmistakable texture and flavor. Follow the recipe step by step, and you will prepare an alternative dish to enjoy with your family.

Prepare the vegetable stock. Coarsely cut a carrot, a peeled potato, a celery rib, and an onion with a drizzle of oil, a pinch of salt and pepper. Leave to cooking for 10 minutes after boiling, then lower the heat to a minimum.

Prepare the vegetables to cook with the meat: cut a carrot, an onion, and a celery rib. Take the turkey breast and tie it with a sprig of rosemary, helping yourself with a string as if it were a roast.

In a large pan, put the turkey to brown in oil with the cut vegetables, a bay leaf, some juniper berries, and a pinch of salt and pepper. Let it brown on all sides turning it gently. At this point, blend with the white wine and let it evaporate. Completely cover the meat and vegetables with the broth and close the pan with a lid. Leave to cook for an hour over a gentle heat until the soup has dried, turn off, and let the meat rest.

Remove the turkey string, slice it with a knife into slices of about one centimeter. Cover them with the tuna sauce. Garnish the turkey with some capers and enjoy it.

Tips

You can store your tuna turkey for up to three days in the fridge.

Recipe 28 - Stew with sirtfood
Serves: 6

Ingredients:

- 1.2 kg beef
- 200 ml red wine
- 80 gr tomato paste
- 4 tablespoons extra virgin olive oil
- 2 garlic cloves
- 1 carrot
- 1 red onion
- 1 celery ribs
- 1 clump of sage
- 1 rosemary sprig
- Broth
- Salt
- Pepper
- Kitchen twine

Directions

The cooking of this recipe is long, but the scents that will be released at home will be worth every wait. Chop the garlic with rosemary and sage, until you have a finely chopped.

Make small cuts on the meat and, using your fingers, insert the chopped meat to flavor the meat. Tie the meat with string so that it keeps its shape while cooking.

Pour the oil and the rest of the chopped vegetables into a saucepan. Insert the piece of meat and brown it slightly. Blend in the red wine and let the alcohol evaporate.

Add the tomato paste. Lower the heat and cook for about 3 hours, until the vegetables are chopped, and the meat is very soft.

Add salt and pepper and serve piping hot.

Recipe 29 – Curly kale with sweet potatoes

Serves: 1

Ingredients:

- 50g Curly Kale
- 200 g Sweet potatoes
- Red onion
- 1 teaspoon bird's eye chilli pepper
- 2 tablespoons extra virgin olive oil
- Salt

Directions

Cut the sweet potatoes into small cubes and put them in a pan with a drizzle of oil and the onion into small pieces. Add salt. Once cooked, add the cut kale and chilli pepper. Turn well until the kale is well withered. Continue cooking for another 5 minutes, always stirring with a ladle!

Recipe 30 – Buckwheat pasta with zucchini and cherry tomatoes

2 servings

Ingredients:

- 160 g buckwheat pasta
- 2 zucchini
- 6 cherry tomatoes
- 1/2 red onion
- extra virgin olive oil
- halls
- bird's-eye chilli

Directions

Fry the oil in a pan with the sliced onion and chilli pepper.

When the onion has taken a little color, add the cherry tomatoes and zucchini slices; turn well and let cook with a lid on medium heat for about 10 minutes, turning occasionally.

Boil the water for the pasta, add salt, and drain the pasta.

Throw it directly into the sauce and fry everything in a pan for about a minute.

Recipe 31 – Chicken curry with potatoes and cabbage

4 servings

Ingredients:

- 600g chicken breast, cut into pieces
- 4 tablespoons of extra virgin olive oil
- 3 tablespoons of turmeric
- 1 red onion, sliced
- 2 red chili peppers, finely chopped
- 2 cloves of garlic, finely chopped
- 1 tablespoon of freshly chopped ginger
- 1 tablespoon curry powder
- 1 jar of cherry tomatoes (400ml)
- 500ml chicken broth
- 200ml of coconut milk
- 2 pieces of cardamom
- 1 cinnamon stick
- 600g potatoes (mostly waxy)
- 10g parsley,
- 175g of kale, cut into pieces,
- 5g of chopped coriander

Marinate the chicken in a teaspoon of olive oil and a tablespoon of turmeric for about 30 minutes.

Fry it in a high frying pan over high heat for about 5 minutes. Remove from the pan and set aside.

Heat a tablespoon of oil in a pan with chilli, garlic, onion, and ginger. Boil over medium heat and then add the curry powder and a tablespoon of turmeric and cook for another minute, stirring occasionally. Add the tomatoes, cook for another two minutes until the chicken stock, coconut milk, cardamom, and cinnamon stick are added. Cook for about 45-60 minutes and add a little broth if necessary. Meanwhile, preheat the oven to 220 °C (425 °F).

Peel and chop the potatoes. Bring the water to the boil, add the potatoes with turmeric and cook for 3 minutes.

Remove them from the water and, in a baking tray, season them with olive oil and curry.Bake in the oven for 30 minutes. When the potatoes and curry are almost ready, add the coriander, cabbage, and chicken and cook for 5 minutes until the chicken is hot.

Add the parsley to the potatoes and serve with the chicken curry.

Recipe 32 – Cabbage and buckwheat soup

1 portion

Ingredients:

- 1 teaspoon of extra virgin olive oil
- 1 teaspoon of mustard seeds
- 1/4 cup (40g) red onion, finely chopped
- 2 cloves of garlic, finely chopped
- 1 teaspoon of finely chopped fresh ginger
- 1 Thai chili pepper, finely chopped
- 1 teaspoon of sweet curry powder, if you prefer)
- 2 teaspoons of ground turmeric
- 300ml vegetable stock or water
- 1/4 cup (40g) Red Lentils, Rinsed
- 3/4 cup (50g) kale, minced
- 50ml canned coconut milk
- 1/3 cup (50g) buckwheat

Directions:

Heat the oil in a medium-sized saucepan over medium heat and add the mustard seeds. When the mustard seeds begin to pop, add the onion, garlic, ginger, and chilli pepper.

Cook for a few minutes. Add the curry powder and one teaspoon of turmeric. After a couple of minutes, add the lentils in the pan and the broth and bring to the boil over low heat for another 25-30 minutes, until the lentils are cooked thoroughly. Add the kale and coconut milk and cook for another 5 minutes. In the meantime, cook the buckwheat according to the package instructions with the remaining teaspoon of turmeric. Drain it and serve it next to the cabbage and lentil soup.

Recipe 33 – Pasta with red chicory and walnuts

Serves: 1

Ingredients:

- 70 g buckwheat pasta
- 100 g red chicory
- 10 g extra virgin olive oil
- 20 g walnuts
- 30 g bacon cut into strips
- 10g Bird's eye chili minced
- Salt

Stew the red chicory in a saucepan with oil, and when it is cooked, add the walnut grains that you have previously browned with bacon cut into strips. In another pot, cook the pasta in salted water, drain it and add it to the mixture of red chicory and walnuts and sauté for a few seconds; finally, a sprinkling of chili.

Recipe 34 - Cabbage and red chicory flan

Serves: 4

Ingredients:

- 800g cabbage
- 250g red chicory
- 100g red onions 100 g
- 3 tablespoons Extra virgin olive oil
- Salt
- Pepper
- 2 tablespoon breadcrumbs
- 60g walnuts

Directions

Clean the cauliflower by eliminating the green leaves and the central core, and always with the help of a smooth blade knife, detach all the tops, dividing in half the bigger ones. Transfer the cleaned buds into a colander and rinse them under cold water.

Put a saucepan full of water on the fire and as soon as it boils, dip the cauliflower tops, cooking them for about 10 minutes; the consistency will have to remain rather al dente, since it will be sautéed in the pan; then continue with the cooking in the oven. Drain the cauliflower into a bowl and leave it aside.

Heat a drizzle of oil in a large pan, add the onion and sauté over low heat. As soon as the onion is golden, add the cauliflower, salt, and pepper to taste. Stir and let everything season for about 5-6 minutes.

In the meantime, clean the red chicory by removing the central core, slice it thinly and add it to the pan with the cauliflower; stir, and fry for a few seconds so as not to wither too much.

Put out the fire and set aside. Chop the nuts.

Heat the oven to 200 °C in static mode. Grease 4 bowls with a diameter of about 11 cm and fill them with cauliflower and red chicory, sprinkle on the surface a pinch of breadcrumbs and walnut grains.

Bake for about 15 minutes, gratinating the last minutes of cooking with the grill to brown the surface. Remove from the oven and serve hot.

You can store the flan in a food container for 2-3 days. We do not recommend freezing.

Recipe 35 - Red chicory and kale salad

Serves: 4

Ingredients:

- 200 g of canned chickpeas
- 1 kale
- 1 red chicory
- 1 red onion
- 40g extra virgin olive oil
- Salt
- Lemon juice
- Walnuts
- Rocket salad

Directions

Clean the kale leaves and cut them into strips. Let them wither with finely chopped red onion in a non-stick pan with two tablespoons of extra virgin olive oil. When the kale is cooked, mix it with the chickpeas, drained from their preserving liquid, in a salad bowl. The ingredient that will give that bitterish touch to the dish will be the red chicory, to be used raw. Mix the various components and then season with fine salt, good extra virgin olive oil, and a splash of lemon, which will give acidity to the dish. Add the walnuts and some arugula leaves to provide color and... enjoy your meal!

Recipe 36 - Salmon and rocket fusilli

Serves: 4

Ingredients:

- 400 g of buckwheat fusilli
- 150 g salmon
- 30 g of fresh ginger
- 80 g arugula
- 1 clove of garlic
- extra virgin olive oil
- Salt
- bird's-eye chili

Directions

To prepare the rocket, salmon and ginger fusilli, put a pot of salted water on the fire. While the pasta is cooking, start making the sauce. Chop the arugula very finely and set it aside. Cut the salmon into cubes and brown it in a pan with a drizzle of oil and crushed garlic until it flakes.

Add the rocket, a few pieces of chili pounded in a mortar, salt, and ginger. Let it all season by stirring. Drain the fusilli well al dente and sauté them in the pan with the seasoning, adding a little cooking water.

Transfer the rocket, salmon and ginger fusilli to the serving plates and serve immediately.

Recipe 37 - Cabbage soup and chickpeas with turmeric

The cabbage and chickpea soup with turmeric is an excellent first course that will warm you up in the autumn season. Healthy and nutritious, thanks to the presence of vegetables and legumes, it is also suitable for those who follow a vegetarian diet.

Coconut milk, so delicate in flavor, harmonizes very well with white cauliflower with a stronger taste, while chickpeas, partly smoothies, give the cream a particular body. Finally, the ginger provides the dish with a spicy note just lively that warms and regenerates, while the turmeric completes the dish with color.

Ingredients:

Serves: 4

- 1 cabbage
- 250 g of chickpeas already cooked
- 400 ml of coconut milk
- 2 teaspoons of turmeric powder
- 1 red onion
- 1 clove of garlic
- 3 cm of freshly grated ginger
- 400 ml hot water
- chopped parsley
- extra virgin olive oil
- salt
- bird's-eye chili

Directions

To prepare the cabbage and chickpea soup with turmeric, start by finely chopping the onion. Brown it in a saucepan with the oil and crushed garlic clove. Add the turmeric, grated ginger, and stir in the onion and let it flavor for a couple of minutes. Add the coconut milk and bring to the boil.

Add the cabbage, cover with water, and cook until tender. Add the chickpeas and let them season for a few minutes. Fill half of the soup to obtain a cream and stir in salt and chilli.

Transfer the cauliflower and chickpeas soup with turmeric to the serving plates and serve with fresh chopped parsley and a round of raw oil to taste.

Recipe 38 - Strawberries in salad

A great dish also suitable for breakfast

Serves: 4

Ingredients:

- 1 head of curly salad
- 150 g strawberries
- 150 g of mixed salads (rocket and soncino)
- extra virgin olive oil
- balsamic vinegar
- salt
- bird's-eye chilli

Directions

Wash and dry the strawberries, remove the stalks, and cut them into slices. Wash the salads, dry them, chop them with your hands. In a salad bowl, pick strawberries and vegetables, stir gently. In a bowl emulsify five tablespoons of oil, two of balsamic vinegar, a pinch of salt, and a few chillies. Drizzle the salad with the sauce, stir and serve.

Recipe 39 - Turmeric chicken

Serves: 4

Ingredients:

- 4 chicken legs
- 4 tablespoons of flour
- 2 tablespoons of turmeric
- 1 red onion
- 20g extra virgin olive oil
- 200 ml of milk
- 4 teaspoons of mustard
- 150 ml of red wine

Directions

Flour the chicken with all powders (keeping a spoonful of turmeric aside).

In a frying pan, cook the sliced onion in oil. Add the chicken and brown it on both sides for a few minutes.

After the red wine has faded, add the milk in which you have dissolved the remaining turmeric.

Cook for 30-40 minutes and before removing from the heat add, if you like, mustard. As for the cooking of the chicken, adjust according to the size and quality of the meat.

Recipe 40 - Pork tenderloin with apricots

Serves: 4

Ingredients:

- 800 gr pork fillet
- 160 gr basmati rice
- 8 apricot
- 3 red onions
- 3 thyme twigs
- 1 rosemary sprig
- 1 teaspoon turmeric
- 2 tablespoons apple vinegar
- 7 tablespoons extra virgin olive oil
- Worcester sauce
- salt
- pepper

Directions

Boil 160 g of basmati rice in plenty of boiling salted water for about 10-12 minutes (or for the time indicated on the package) and drain it al dente. Place it in a bowl and smell it with 1 teaspoon of turmeric.

Put in a glass jar 6 tablespoons of extra virgin olive oil, two tablespoons of apple vinegar, salt, and pepper, close with the lid and shake vigorously, to emulsify.

Prepare the other ingredients. While the rice is boiling, peel two red onions, cut them into large slices, cook them on the grill for 5 minutes on each side; arrange them in a baking dish and keep them warm in the oven at 180° C. Wash, dry, and cut eight apricots in half without the stone, and cook them on the grill for 5 minutes on each side. Also, transfer the apricots to the baking tray.

Cut 800 g of pork fillet into 2.5 cm thick slices, to make the meat tastier; leave the slices to rest for 20 minutes in a marinade made with one tablespoon of extra virgin olive oil, chopped onion, thyme, rosemary, and Worchestershire sauce.

Complete and serve. Cook the meat on the steak for about 6 minutes on each side. If needed, transfer the slices to a heat-resistant serving plate and keep them warm for a few minutes in the oven. When everything is ready, season the ingredients with the apple vinegar vinaigrette and serve at the table, accompanying the apricot pork tenderloin with the turmeric-scented rice.

CHAPTER 9: QUESTIONS & ANSWERS

1. **Should I exercise during the first phase?**

   Regular exercise is essential for health, and moderate physical activity will increase weight loss and the benefits of the first stage of the diet. But listen to your body. There is no need to stress yourself with intense or prolonged sports activities during the first phase; let the Sirt foods do the work a bit.

2. **I'm obese. Is the Sirt diet suitable for me?**

   Yes, it is. According to studies on the activity of sirtuins, you should reap the maximum benefits not only in terms of weight loss but also in terms of general well-being. Obesity increases the risk of suffering from chronic diseases, the same illnesses that Sirt foods help to protect you from.

3. **I'm sporty. Can I go on the Sirt diet too?**

   Yes. Sirt foods have become a winning strategy for many sports champions, allowing them to achieve their goals in terms of body composition and, more generally, fitness.

4. **I want to lose fat but not muscle mass and tone, is that possible?**

Yes, the type of slimming of the Sirt diet is just that. In any other diet, if someone loses 3.5 kg per week, at least 900 grams is muscle. Sirt foods, on the other hand, activate not only fat consumption, but also promote muscle growth and repair. It means that you not only lose weight, but you also look better and more toned.

5. **Can I eat all the Sirt foods I want, even high-calorie foods, and lose weight anyway?**

   Yes! Thanks to the effects on your metabolism and appetite, you don't have to worry about eating too many Sirt foods. We don't invite you to binge but eat these foods until you feel full. The only exception are dates. When it comes to beverages, the consumption of red wine must be in moderation, but this is obvious to everyone, responsible.

6. **It all seems too "miraculous" to me. Will you also tell me that I'll live longer?**

   Yes, in a certain way, sirtuins are miracles of nature, because they regulate the metabolism of our body. And yes, it has been scientifically proven that in cultures where you eat more Sirt food, the incidence of cancer is lower. Heart disease, diabetes, dementia, and osteoporosis are just some of the conditions that can be prevented by activating sirtuins.

7. **I'm already skinny. Can I follow this diet?**

   If you're underweight, you should avoid phase 1. Although it is understandable to want to be even thinner, going beyond the point of being underweight is incredibly unhealthy, both physically and mentally. While a person who is overweight or well within a healthy weight can practice stage 1, no one who is clinically underweight should do so. You can still introduce t-shirt foods into your diet to receive the benefits that sirtuins have to offer.

8. **Can I drink red wine during the first phase?**

   It is not recommendable to drink alcohol during the first phase. However, you can drink it in moderation during phase two and the maintenance phase.

Conclusion

Dear reader, thank you for coming all the way to the end of this book. I hope you enjoyed it, but most of all, that you will be able to benefit from it. When I started this diet, I didn't think it could be that effective because I had tried so many dietary plans in the past without success.

Many times we believe that we are condemned to live always in the same way, but each of us can be able to change our lives. Remember that slimming should not be lived only as a race. The goal is to find your body, your image, your beauty, your health, your life, your physical condition, and the pride of being the conductor of your body to be able to direct it and not suffer it passively.

I have a hard life, but I have decided to devote part of my time to writing this book so that others can finally change the relationship with their bodies and their health.

Thank you, and a happy change of life to you!

Conversions

Grams to Ounces

1 gram (g) is equal to 0.03527396195 ounces (oz).

Formula:

| 1 g = 0.03527396195 oz |

The mass y in ounces (oz) is equal to the mass y in grams (g) divided by 28.34952:

$y_{(oz)} =$ $y_{(g)} / \mathbf{28.34952}$

Example

Convert 100g to Ounces:

$y_{(oz)} =$ 100 g / 28.34952 = 3,5274 oz

Table

Grams (g)	Ounces (oz)
0 g	0 oz
1 g	0.0353 oz
2 g	0.0706 oz
3 g	0.1058 oz
4 g	0.1411 oz
5 g	0.1764 oz
6 g	0.2116 oz
7 g	0.2469 oz
8 g	0.2822 oz
9 g	0.3175 oz
10 g	0.3527 oz
20 g	0.7055 oz
30 g	1.0582 oz

40 g	1.4110 oz
50 g	1.7637 oz
60 g	2.1164 oz
70 g	2.4692 oz
80 g	2.8219 oz
90 g	3.1747 oz
100 g	3.5274 oz
1000 g	35.2740 oz

Celsius to Fahrenheit

0 grade Celsius (°C) is equal to 32 Fahrenheit (°F)
1 grade Celsius (°C) is equal to 33.8 F Fahrenheit (°F)

Formula:

$$(n\ °C \times 9/5) + 32 = n\ °F$$

Example

Convert 200 °C to °F
(200 x 9/5)+32= 392 °F

Table

Celsius (°C)	Fahrenheit (°F)
0	32
60	140
70	158
80	176
90	194
100	212
110	230
120	248
130	266
140	284
150	302
160	320
170	338
180	356
190	374
200	392
210	410
220	428

Printed in Great Britain
by Amazon